Renal Physiology

Second Edition

Arthur J. Vander, M.D.
Professor of Physiology
University of Michigan

McGraw-Hill Book Company

New York St. Louis San Francisco Auckland Bogotá Hamburg
Johannesburg London Madrid Mexico Montreal New Delhi
Panama Paris São Paulo Singapore Sydney Tokyo Toronto

RENAL PHYSIOLOGY

567890 HDHD 898765432

This book was set in Times Roman by The Clarinda Company.
The editors were Richard W. Mixter and Abe Krieger;
the production supervisor was Robert A. Pirrung.
The drawings were done by J & R Services, Inc.
The cover was designed by Antonia Goldmark.

Library of Congress Cataloging in Publication Data

Vander, Arthur J   date
   Renal physiology.

   Bibliography: p.
   Includes index.
   1. Kidneys. I. Title. [DNLM: 1. Kidney—Physiology.
WJ300.3 V228r]
QP249.V36   1980   612'.463   79-18428
ISBN 0-07-066958-9

Contents

Preface

This book is my attempt to identify the essential core content of renal physiology appropriate for medical students and to present it in a way which permits the student to master the material independently, i.e., with no (or very few) accompanying lectures by the instructor. I have been gratified by the wide use the first edition has achieved and the many letters I have received from medical students (and clinicians) who found they were, indeed, able to master its contents by independent study.

Accordingly, my major goals in preparing this edition have been to update the material thoroughly and to strive for greater clarity of exposition (to this latter end, a large number of new flow diagrams has been added) but not to alter the level of coverage. There is one major exception to this last guideline; I have added a systematic description (in Chap. 2) of the general categories of transport processes and their interactions in achieving transepithelial transport and have then applied these concepts to specific solutes in later chapters. I have also expanded the sections on the transport of urea and organic acids and bases. The task of sticking to my intent of presenting only core material was even more painful this time because of the explosion of information in renal physiology over the past 4 years. I can only plead once again with my fellow teachers to share with me their views concerning my choice.

My selection of this core material is made explicit in a comprehensive list of behavioral objectives, which tell students specifically what I believe they should know and be able to do by the book's completion. Obviously, no two instructors would come up with exactly the same core material, but it is a simple matter for instructors to give students a supplementary list of goals to be added or deleted. The information required to achieve any additional goals not covered in the book would, of course, have to be provided by other reading assignments or lectures. However, my belief, based on consultations with other physiologists and clinicians, is that these discrepancies are likely to be few. Of much greater importance is the fact that the behavioral goals (in essence, the content of the book) are explicitly defined so that any such differences are easily determined. This also makes the book quite usable for students in other health sciences, whose required core of information might differ from that of medical students.

In addition to the comprehensive objectives, I have included a large number of study questions with annotated answers. Unlike the lists of objectives, the study questions are neither systematic nor comprehensive in their coverage. Rather, they generally deal with areas I have found usually difficult for students and give them practice and additional feedback.

I advise the student to go through the book one chapter at a time. Some students profit by using the objectives to guide their readings as they proceed through a chapter. In any case, at the end of each chapter go over the objectives in detail and the study questions (at the back of the book) relevant to that chapter. They provide you with the means for determining whether you have mastered the material and for identifying those specific areas which require more work.

I should like to point out several characteristics of the book common to most texts but particularly common in this type of book. I have rarely included the original research upon which this core of knowledge rests, nor have I been able to explore the fascinating controversies in virtually every area. Therefore, the Suggested Readings at the back of the book are of considerable importance for the student who wishes to pursue any subject in greater depth. They are almost all review articles, and their bibliographies provide an entry into the original research literature. The question of how to handle controversy in such a book is a particularly perplexing one. I have tried to present various views (frequently in footnotes) in areas where the evidence is closely balanced, but I have often simply had to ignore an opposing view. Obviously, such decisions are always arbitrary, to a large degree, and I can only apologize, in advance, to those of my colleagues who feel I have slighted their work.

Finally, I should like to thank Peggy Rogers for her splendid typing of the manuscript.

Arthur J. Vander

Chapter 1

Function and Structure
of the Kidneys

OBJECTIVES

The student states the balance concept.

The student knows the functions of the kidneys.
1 Lists seven functions
2 States the components of the renin-angiotensin system and their biochemical interrelations
3 States the role of renal erythropoietic factor

The student defines important gross structures and knows their interrelationships: renal pelvis, calyxes, renal pyramids, medulla, cortex, papilla

The student understands the interrelationships between the components of a nephron.
1 Defines glomerulus and tubule
2 Draws the relationship between glomerular capillaries, Bowman's capsule, and the proximal tubule
3 States the three layers separating the lumen of the glomerular capillaries and Bowman's space; defines podocytes, foot processes, slits, and slit diaphragms

4 Lists in order all the tubular segments; defines proximal tubule, loop of Henle, distal tubule, and collecting duct in physiologists' convention
5 Describes the differences between outer cortical and inner cortical (juxtamedullary) nephrons
6 Defines interstitial cells
7 Defines juxtaglomerular apparatus and states the relationship between its components

The student understands the blood supply to the nephron.
1 Lists, in order, the vessels through which blood flows from renal artery to renal vein
2 Defines vasa recta

FUNCTIONS

Regulation of Water and Electrolyte Balance

A cell's function depends not only upon receiving a continuous supply of nutrients and eliminating its metabolic end products but also upon the existence of stable physicochemical conditions in the extracellular fluid bathing it, Claude Bernard's "internal environment." Maintenance of this stability is the primary function of the kidneys.

Since the extracellular fluid occupies an intermediate position between the external environment and the cells, the concentration of any substance within it can be altered by exchange in either direction. Exchanges with cells are called *internal exchanges*. For example, a decrease in extracellular potassium concentration is followed by a counteracting movement of potassium out of cells into the extracellular fluid. Each type of ion is stored in cells or in bone in significant amounts, which can be partially depleted or expanded without damage to the storage site. But these stores are limited, and in the long run any deficit or excess of total body water or total body electrolyte must be compensated by exchanges with the external environment, i.e., by changes in intake or output.

A substance appears in the body either as a result of ingestion or as a product of metabolism. Conversely, a substance can be excreted from the body or consumed in a metabolic reaction. Therefore, if the quantity of any substance in the body is to be maintained at a constant level over a period of time, the total amounts ingested and produced must equal the total amounts excreted and consumed. This is a general statement of the *balance concept*. For water and hydrogen ion all four possible pathways apply. However, balance is simpler for the mineral electrolytes. Since they are neither synthesized nor consumed by cells, their total body balance reflects only ingestion versus excretion.

As an example, let us describe the balance for total body water (Table 1). It should be recognized that these are average values, which are sub-

Table 1 Normal Routes of Water Gain and Loss in Adults

Route	mL/day
Intake	
Drunk	1200
In food	1000
Metabolically produced	350
Total	2550
Output	
Insensible loss (skin and lungs)	900
Sweat	50
In feces	100
Urine	1500
Total	2550

ject to considerable variation. The two sources of body water are metabolically produced water, resulting largely from the oxidation of carbohydrates, and ingested water, obtained from liquids and so-called solid food (a rare steak is approximately 70 percent water).

There are four sites from which water is lost to the external environment: skin, lungs, gastrointestinal tract, and kidneys. The loss of water by evaporation from the cells of the skin and the lining of respiratory passageways is a continuous process, often referred to as *insensible loss* because the person is unaware of its occurrence. Additional water can be made available for evaporation from the skin by the production of sweat.

Under normal conditions, as can be seen from the table, water loss exactly equals water gain, and no net change of body water occurs. This is obviously no accident but the result of precise regulatory mechanisms. The question then is: Which processes involved in water balance are controlled to make the gains and losses balance? The answer, as we shall see, is voluntary intake *(thirst)* and urinary loss. This does not mean that none of the other processes is controlled, but it does mean their control is not primarily oriented toward water balance. Carbohydrate catabolism, the major source of water from oxidation, is controlled by mechanisms directed toward regulation of energy balance. Sweat production is controlled by mechanisms directed toward temperature regulation. Insensible loss in humans is truly uncontrolled. Fecal water loss is generally unchanging and is normally quite small (but can be severe in vomiting or diarrhea).

The mechanism of thirst is certainly of great importance, since body deficits of water, regardless of cause, must be made up by ingestion of water. But it is also true that our fluid intake is often influenced more by habit and by sociological factors than by the need to regulate body water. The control of urinary water loss is the major automatic mechanism by which body water is regulated.

By similar analyses, we find that the body balances of many of the ions determining the properties of the extracellular fluid are regulated primarily by the kidneys. To appreciate the importance of these kidney regulations one need only make a partial list of the more important simple inorganic substances which constitute the internal environment and which are regulated in large part by the kidneys: water, sodium, potassium, chloride, calcium, magnesium, sulfate, phosphate, and hydrogen ion. Indeed, the extraordinary number of substances which the kidney regulates and the precision with which these processes normally occur accounted for the kidneys being the last stronghold of the nineteenth century vitalists, who simply would not believe that the laws of physics and chemistry could fully explain renal function. By what mechanism does urine flow rapidly increase when a person ingests several glasses of liquid? How is it that the patient on an extremely low salt intake and the person who eats a great deal of salt both urinate precisely the amounts of salt required to maintain their sodium balance? What mechanisms decrease the urinary calcium excretion of children deprived of milk?

Excretion of Metabolic Waste Products

The regulatory role just described is obviously quite different from the popular conception of the kidneys as glorified garbage disposal units which rid the body of assorted wastes and poisons. It is true that some of the chemical reactions which occur within cells result ultimately in end products that must be eliminated. These end products are called waste products because they serve no known biological function in humans. For example, the catabolism of protein produces approximately 30 g of urea per day. Other end products produced in relatively large quantities are uric acid (from nucleic acids), creatinine (from muscle creatine), bilirubin and other end products of hemoglobin breakdown, and the metabolites of various hormones. There are many others, not all of which have been completely identified. Most of these substances are eliminated from the body as rapidly as they are produced, primarily by way of the kidneys. Some of them, e.g., urea, are relatively harmless, but the accumulation of others within the body during periods of renal malfunction accounts for some of the disordered body functions in the patient suffering from severe kidney disease. We still are not sure as to the identity of these "toxins" or which of the problems occurring in renal disease are due to them, as opposed to disordered water-and-electrolyte metabolism.

Excretion of Foreign Chemicals

The kidneys have another excretory function, which is presently assuming increasing importance, namely, the elimination from the body of foreign chemicals, such as drugs, pesticides, food additives, and their metabolites.

Regulation of Arterial Blood Pressure

The kidneys are intimately involved in the regulation of arterial blood pressure by several mechanisms.

First, sodium balance is a critical determinant of cardiac output (and, possibly, arteriolar resistance, over any long time period), and the kidneys, as stated above, regulate this balance.

Second, the kidneys function as endocrine glands in the *renin-angiotensin system,* a hormonal complex of enzymes, proteins, and peptides which are importantly involved in the regulation of arterial pressure. *Renin* is a proteolytic enzyme secreted into the blood by the kidneys, specifically by the granular cells of the juxtaglomerular apparatuses (see below). Once in the bloodstream, renin catalyzes the splitting of a decapeptide, *angiotensin I,* from a plasma protein known as *angiotensinogen,* which is secreted by the liver and is always present in the plasma in high concentration. Under the influence of another enzyme, *converting enzyme,* the terminal two amino acids are then split from the relatively inactive angiotensin I to yield the octapeptide *angiotensin II.* Converting enzyme is present in plasma and in many organs but is most concentrated in the endothelial cells lining the pulmonary capillaries; accordingly, the conversion of angiotensin I to angiotensin II occurs mainly as blood flows through lung capillaries. Until recently it was assumed that angiotensin II is the only physiologically active peptide in the system. However, as Fig. 1 illustrates, angiotensin II can be split to yield the heptapeptide known as

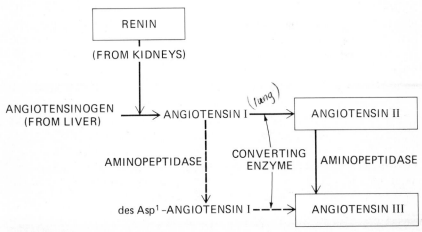

Figure 1 Basic biochemistry of renin-angiotensin system. The solid arrows denote the major pathway, the dashed arrows a possible alternate pathway for the generation of angiotensin III.

angiotensin III, and it is almost certain that this latter peptide is also quite active biologically. (The enzymes which mediate its generation seem to be located mainly in the target tissues for this peptide.) An evaluation of the relative contributions of antiotensin II or III (angiotensin I does not exert significant effects) to the effects of the overall system is beyond the scope of this book, and we shall simply refer to these peptides collectively as angiotensin.[1] As we shall see in subsequent chapters, angiotensin exerts an immense number of effects on diverse tissues, but the end results of most of them are to increase arterial blood pressure. A crucial generalization to be gained from the biochemistry of this system is that because angiotensinogen and the enzymes beyond renin are usually present in relatively unchanging concentration,[2] the primary determinant of the rate of angiotensin formation is the plasma concentration of renin, which is physiologically regulated via the control of renin secretion.

In addition to their regulation of salt balance and secretion of renin, the kidneys may exert a third important influence over arterial blood pressure. It is very likely that they either secrete into the blood or remove from it vasoactive substances other than renin. Certainly the kidneys are capable of synthesizing a number of prostaglandins, both vasodilator and vasoconstrictor in action, and the possibility that one or more of these prostaglandins may reach the systemic arterial blood in amounts adequate to dilate or constrict arterioles is the subject of considerable investigation. Lipids other than prostaglandins have also been implicated in the renal regulation of arterial blood pressure.

Regulation of Erythrocyte Production

The kidneys secrete a second hormone, *renal erythropoietic factor* (REF), which is involved in the control of erythrocyte production by the bone marrow. Just which renal cells secrete REF is not yet clear, but the stimulus for its secretion is a decrease in oxygen delivery to the kidneys (as, for example, in anemia, hypoxia, or hypotension with inadequate renal blood flow). Once secreted, REF acts enzymatically in the plasma on a globulin (secreted by the liver) to split off a polypeptide known as erythropoietin, which then stimulates the bone marrow to increase its production of erythrocytes. (Note the analogies between the biochemistry of this system and that of the renin-angiotensin system.) The REF-

---

[1]The renin-angiotensin system is among the most intensively studied fields in the medical sciences, and its biochemistry grows more bewildering every day as "prorenins," "pseudorenins," "brain renins," alternate pathways, etc. accumulate. The reader interested in going beyond the extremely basic descriptions given in this book should consult the Suggested Readings.

[2]There are clinically important situations in which changes in angiotensinogen or converting enzyme may significantly influence the generation of angiotensin. For example, oral contraceptives may cause a large increase in plasma angiotensinogen.

erythropoietin system will not be described further in this book; suffice it to say that renal disease may result in diminished REF secretion, and the ensuing decrease in bone marrow activity is one important causal factor in the anemia of chronic renal disease.

Regulation of Vitamin D Activity

The kidneys produce the active form of vitamin D (1,25-dihydroxyvitamin D_3). This makes the third hormone secreted by the kidneys; its synthesis and role in calcium metabolism will be described in Chap. 10.

Gluconeogenesis

During prolonged fasting, the kidneys synthesize glucose from amino acids and other precursors and release it into the blood. Thus, like the liver, they are gluconeogenic organs.

STRUCTURE OF THE KIDNEYS AND URINARY SYSTEM

The kidneys are paired organs which lie outside the peritoneal cavity in the posterior abdominal wall, one on each side of the vertebral column. The medial border of the kidney is indented by a deep fissure (called the hilum) through which passes the renal vessels and nerves and in which lies the funnel-shaped continuation of the upper end of the ureter, the *renal pelvis* (Fig. 2). The outer convex border of the renal pelvis is divided into major *calyxes*, each of which subdivides into several minor calyxes. Each of the latter is cupped around the projecting apex of a cone-shaped mass of tissue *(a renal pyramid)*.

When the kidney is bisected from top to bottom it can be seen to be divided into two major regions: an inner *renal medulla* and an outer *renal cortex*. The medulla is made up of a number of renal pyramids, the apexes of which, as stated above, project into the minor calyxes. Each pyramid of the medulla, topped by a region of renal cortex, forms a single lobe.

Upon closer gross examination, additional features can be discerned: (1) The cortex has a highly granular appearance missing from the medulla; (2) each medullary pyramid is divisible into an outer zone (adjacent to the cortex) and an inner zone, including the apical tip, called the *papilla*. All these distinctions reflect the arrangement of the various components of the microscopic subunits of the kidneys, to which we now turn.

The Nephron

In humans, each kidney is composed of approximately 1 million tiny units, *nephrons,* one of which is shown diagrammatically in Fig. 3. Each nephron consists of a "filtering component," called the *glomerulus,* and a

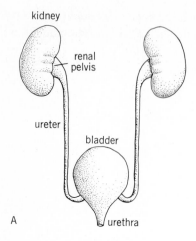

A

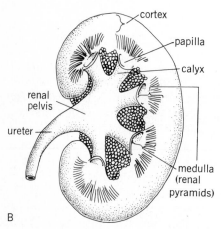

B

Figure 2 A. The urinary system. The urine, formed by the kidney, collects in the renal pelvis and then flows through the ureter into the bladder, from which it is eliminated via the urethra. B. Section of a human kidney. Half the kidney has been sliced away. Note that the structure shows regional differences. The outer portion (cortex), which has a granular appearance, contains all the glomeruli. The collecting ducts form a large portion of the inner kidney (medulla), giving it a striped, pyramidlike appearance, and drain into the renal pelvis. The papilla is the inner portion of the medulla. *(From A. J. Vander et al., Human Physiology, © 1970 by McGraw-Hill, Inc. Used with permission of McGraw-Hill Book Company.)*

tubule extending out from the glomerulus. Let us begin with the glomerulus, which is responsible for the initial step in urine formation, the separation of a protein-free filtrate from plasma.

The Glomerulus   The glomerulus consists of a compact tuft of interconnected capillary loops (the *glomerular capillaries*) and a balloonlike hollow capsule *(Bowman's capsule)* into which the capillary tuft protrudes (Fig. 4).[1] One way of visualizing the relationship between the glomerular capillaries and Bowman's capsule is to imagine a loosely clenched fist (the capillaries) punched into a balloon (Bowman's capsule).

---

[1]There is no complete agreement as to whether the glomerulus should refer only to the capillary tuft or to the tuft plus Bowman's capsule; the latter is presently the more common usage.

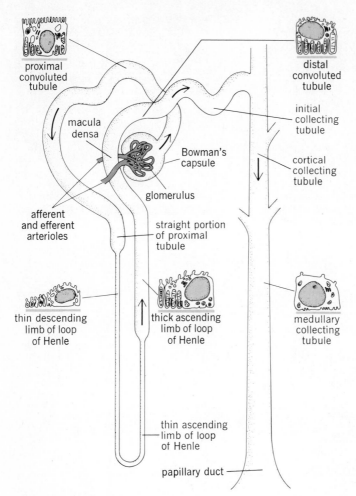

Figure 3 Relationships of component parts of the nephron, which has been "uncoiled" for clarity; relative lengths of the different segments are not accurate. [*Drawings of fine structure adapted from J. Rhodin, Int. Rev. Cytol., 7:485 (1958).*]

The part of Bowman's capsule in contact with the glomerular capillaries becomes pushed inward but does not make contact with the opposite side of the capsule; accordingly, a space *(Bowman's space)* still exists within the capsule, and it is into this space that fluid filters from the glomerular capillaries across the combined capillary–Bowman's capsule membranes.

This filtration barrier consists of three layers: capillary endothelium, basement membrane, and the single-celled layer of capsular epithelial cells (Fig. 4). The first layer, the endothelial cells of the capillaries, is perforated by many large fenestrae. The basement membrane is a relatively

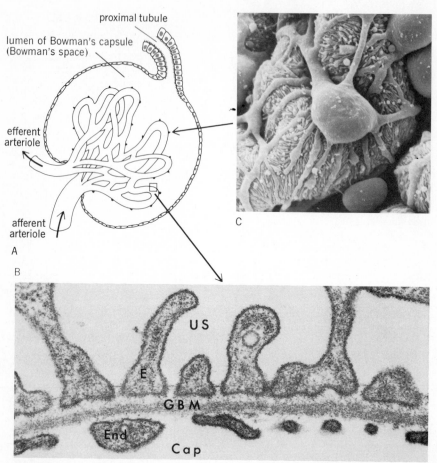

Figure 4   A. Anatomy of the glomerulus. B. Cross section of glomerular membranes US = "Urinary" (Bowman's) space, E = epithelial foot processes, GBM = glomerular basement membranes, End = capillary endothelium, Cap = lumen of capillary. Note the basement membrane is itself not homogenous but has a denser core. [*Courtesy H. G. Rennke; originally published in Fed. Proc.* **36:**2619 (1977); *reprinted with permission.*] C. Scanning electron micrograph of podocytes covering glomerular capillary loops; the view is from inside Bowman's space. The large mass is a cell body. Note the remarkable interdigitation of the foot processes from adjacent podocytes and the slits between them. *(Courtesy of Dr. Craig Tisher.)*

homogenous acellular meshwork of glycoproteins and mucopolysaccharides. The epithelial cells in this region of the glomerulus are quite different from the relatively simple, flattened cells lining the rest of Bowman's capsule (the part of the "balloon" not in contact with the "fist") and are called *podocytes;* they have an unusual octopuslike structure in that they possess a large number of extensions, or *foot processes,* which are embedded in the basement membrane, foot processes from adjacent podocytes manifesting a great degree of interdigitation. *Slits* exist between adjacent foot processes and constitute the path through which the filtrate, once through the endothelial cells and basement membrane, travels to enter Bowman's space. However, for two reasons, these slits do not offer completely open passageways: (1) The foot processes are coated by a thick layer of extracellular material (glycosialoproteins), which partially occludes the slits; (2) extremely thin diaphragms bridge the slits at the surface of the basement membrane.

The functional significance of this anatomical arrangement is that blood in the glomerular capillaries is separated from Bowman's space only by a thin set of membranes, which permits the filtration of fluid from the capillaries into the space. Bowman's capsule connects at the side opposite the glomerular tuft with the first portion of the tubule, into which this filtered fluid then flows.

The Tubule   Throughout its course, the tubule is composed of a single layer of epithelial cells resting on a basement membrane. The structure of these epithelial cells varies considerably from segment to segment, but one common feature is the presence of tight junctions between adjacent cells.

The segment of the tubule which drains Bowman's capsule is the *proximal tubule* (Fig. 3), which initially forms several coils (the convoluted portion of the proximal tubule) followed by a relatively straight segment. There are structural differences between the convoluted and straight portions of the proximal tubule, and functional heterogeneity may also exist; however, we shall treat them as a single nephron segment (Table 2).

Table 2   Terms Used to Denote Tubular Segments*

Combination terms traditionally used by anatomists	Sequence of distinct tubular segments	Combination terms traditionally used by physiologists
Proximal tubule	Proximal convoluted tubule Proximal straight tubule	Proximal tubule
Loop of Henle	Thin descending limb of Henle's loop Thin ascending limb of Henle's loop Thick ascending limb of Henle's loop	Loop of Henle
Distal tubule	Macula densa Distal convoluted tubule	Distal tubule
Collecting ducts	Initial collecting tubule Cortical collecting tubule Medullary collecting tubule Papillary duct	Collecting duct

*Individual tubules begin to join with each other at the level of the cortical collecting tubules. The sequence given in the central column is by no means exhaustive, for subdivisions of several of the segments are identifiable and have been given separate names, but these are not yet in common use. (To add to the complexity, not all nephrons have all the segments listed in the central column.) Finally, it is helpful to recognize that physiologists often refer to "early" and "late" distal tubule, signifying distal convoluted tubule and initial collecting tubule, respectively.

The next portion of the tubule is a sharp hairpinlike loop called the *loop of Henle*. Throughout its entire length, the *descending limb of the loop* is quite thin. At the hairpin turn, the *ascending limb* begins, and a transition occurs in the epithelium. In long loops, the first portion of the ascending limb remains thin (but different from the descending limb), and the upper portion, then, becomes thick; in short loops, the entire ascending limb is thick (Fig. 5).

At the end of the ascending limb of Henle's loop, the tubule passes between the arterioles supplying its glomerulus of origin (Fig. 3), and this very short segment is known as the *macula densa*. Beyond the macula densa, the tubule once more becomes coiled as the *distal convoluted tubule*, which empties into an *initial collecting tubule*. From the glomerulus to the end of the initial collecting tubule, each of the 1 million

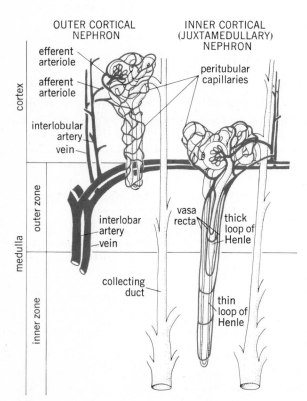

Figure 5 Comparison of the blood supplies of outer cortical and juxtamedullary nephrons. This figure is misleading in one regard in that it suggests that the peritubular capillaries of a tubule are derived only from the efferent arteriole leaving that tubule's glomerulus of origin; in fact, they are derived from efferent arterioles coming from many glomeruli. *(Redrawn from R. F. Pitts, Physiology of the Kidney and Body Fluids, 3d ed., Year Book, Chicago, 1974.)*

tubules is completely separate from the others. Multiple initial collecting tubules from separate nephrons join to form *cortical collecting tubules,* which then turn downward to enter the medulla. Now called *medullary collecting tubules,* they finally empty into a calyx of the renal pelvis, the very last portion being termed a papillary duct. The calyx is continuous with the *ureter,* which empties into the *urinary bladder,* where urine is temporarily stored and from which it is intermittently eliminated. The urine is not altered after it enters a calyx. From this point on, the remainder of the urinary system simply serves as plumbing.

Physiologists and anatomists have traditionally grouped two or more continuous tubular segments for purposes of reference, but unfortunately the terminologies used in these disciplines have not been identical. Table 2 summarizes these terms. Combination terms used in this book will follow the physiologists' convention.

Blood Supply to the Nephrons

In the earlier section on the glomerulus, we described the glomerular capillaries but made no mention of their origin. Blood enters each kidney via a renal artery, which then divides into progressively smaller branches. Each of the smallest arteries of the cortex (the interlobular arteries) gives off at right angles to itself, as it courses toward the kidney surface, a parallel series of *afferent arterioles* (Figs. 3 and 5), each of which leads to a glomerulus. (Thus, the afferent arteriole is the "arm" to which the "fist" is attached.)

Normally, only about 20 percent of the plasma (and none of the erythrocytes) entering the glomerular capillaries is filtered into Bowman's capsule; where does the remaining blood go next? In almost all other organs, capillaries recombine to form the beginnings of the venous system. The glomerular capillaries instead recombine to form another set of arterioles called the *efferent arterioles.* Thus, blood leaves the glomerulus through an arteriole, which soon subdivides into a second set of capillaries (Fig. 5). These *peritubular capillaries* are profusely distributed to, and intimately associated with, all the portions of the tubule, an arrangement which permits movement of solutes and water between the tubular lumen and capillaries. They rejoin to form the venous channels by which blood ultimately leaves the kidney.

Regional Differences in Structure

There are important regional differences in the locations of the various tubular and vascular components. The cortex contains all the glomeruli (this accounts for its granular appearance), proximal and distal tubules, cortical collecting tubules, and portions of the loops of Henle. In humans, approximately 90 percent of the nephrons originate in glomeruli located in the superficial and intermediate areas of the cortex and have relatively short loops of Henle, which may extend only into the outer medulla; they are known as *outer cortical nephrons*. The remaining 10 percent originate in glomeruli located in the innermost, or *juxtamedullary, cortex* (i.e., "cortex just adjacent to the medulla"). These so-called *juxtamedullary nephrons,* in contrast to the outer cortical nephrons, have long loops, which extend deep into the medulla, where they run parallel to the collecting ducts; note (Fig. 5) that the additional length of the loop of Henle in juxtamedullary nephrons is due entirely to the long thin segment. (The beginning of the thick ascending limb in the longest loops marks the border between outer and inner medulla.)

The outer cortical and juxtamedullary nephrons differ from each other structurally in many ways other than the lengths of their loops of Henle; moreover, the outer cortical nephrons themselves are not homogenous but manifest gradations of structural characteristics as one moves inward from the cortical surface. It seems certain that this structural heterogeneity is also reflected in functional heterogeneity.

The vascular structures supplying the juxtamedullary nephrons also differ in that their efferent arterioles drain not only into the usual peritubular-capillary network of the cortex and outer medulla but also into thin hairpin-loop vessels *(vasa recta),* which run parallel to the loops of Henle and collecting ducts in the inner medulla; this arrangement has considerable significance for renal function, as will be described later.

One other regional difference concerns the so-called interstitial cells, which become more numerous and larger as one descends from cortex to papilla. These cells, which are located between adjacent tubules and capillaries, are thought to synthesize and release prostaglandins in response to appropriate stimuli.

The Juxtaglomerular Apparatus

Reference was made earlier to the macula densa, that portion of the tubule which marks the transition between the ascending loop of Henle and the distal convoluted tubule. In all nephrons, this segment courses between the afferent and efferent arterioles at their points of contact with the glomerulus of the macula densa's own nephron. This area of contact is known as the *juxtaglomerular (JG) apparatus*. (Don't confuse the term "juxtaglomerular apparatus" with "juxtamedullary nephron.") Each JG apparatus is composed of three cell types: (1) *granular cells,* which appear to be differentiated smooth muscle cells in the walls of the arterioles (particularly in the afferent arterioles); (2) so-called mesangial cells, which have an uncertain origin; and (3) the macula densa cells. The granular cells are the cells which secrete the hormone renin, mentioned earlier in this chapter. The macula densa, via its intimate contact with the granular cells, contributes to the control of renin secretion, as will be described in

Chap. 7. The juxtaglomerular apparatus may also offer a pathway for controlling renal hemodynamics via a nonrenin mechanism (see Chap. 5).

METHODS IN RENAL PHYSIOLOGY

Because of its scope and objectives, this book will deal very little with the methods used to generate the content of renal physiology. Only the method known as "clearance" is described to any extent (in Chap. 4) because of its widespread clinical use. The other technique which has been the mainstay of renal physiologists is *micropuncture*, the insertion of a micropipette into a nephron segment and withdrawal of fluid for analysis. This technique was originally established by A. N. Richards and his collaborators for use in amphibians, whose nephrons are relatively large and can be seen easily since they are not packed together into an enclosed organ. Micropuncture has since been used to withdraw fluid from nephron segments of mammalian kidneys, as well as to measure pressures, perfuse tubules, and perform other manipulations on single nephrons in situ. More recently, a technique has been developed for perfusing isolated separated segments of a single nephron in vitro, and this is making possible many studies previously closed to micropuncture.[1]

In addition to clearance, micropuncture, and the isolated, perfused tubule, a plethora of other useful techniques has been developed, and all of them, like the "big three," have particular advantages and disadvantages. The interested reader should consult the list of Suggested Readings at the back of the book.

Study questions: **1** and **2**

[1]For example, micropuncture is generally applicable only to the outermost nephrons since these can be visualized by looking down upon the surface of the kidney. This has been a major impediment to studying functional nephron heterogeneity.

Chapter 2

Basic Renal Processes

OBJECTIVES

The student knows the basic principles of renal physiology.
1 Lists and defines the three renal processes: glomerular filtration, tubular reabsorption, tubular secretion
2 Describes the routes for blood and fluid movements within the kidneys
3 Describes the chemical characteristics of the glomerular filtrate
4 States the sites in the glomerulus for restriction of macromolecules; defines steric hindrance and electrical hindrance and relates them to protein filtration
5 States the formula for the determinants of glomerular net filtration pressure and the normal values for each determinant
6 Predicts the direction of change of GFR under a variety of situations, including hypotension, reduced plasma protein concentration, and ureteral occlusion
7 Describes the method and formula used for measurement of GFR and states its normal value
8 Defines and states the major characteristics of simple facilitated diffusion, coupled facilitated diffusion (and secondary active transport), primary active transport, and endocytosis

9 States how the mechanisms of objective 8 can be combined to achieve net transepithelial movement (i.e., net reabsorption or secretion); diagrams the pathways for reabsorption of sodium and glucose

10 Defines the concept of T_m (either reabsorptive or secretory); given appropriate data, calculates T_m; defines splay and describes the mechanism for it; states the significance of a T_m being much higher than the usual filtered mass of the substance

11 States the two major types of carrier-mediated systems for secretion of organic solutes by the proximal tubule

12 Defines "pump-leak" system and states its consequences

Urine formation begins with the filtration of essentially protein-free plasma through the glomerular capillaries into Bowman's capsule. The final urine which enters the renal pelvis is quite different from the *glomerular filtrate* because, as the filtered fluid flows from Bowman's capsule through the various portions of the tubule, its composition is altered. This change occurs by two general processes: tubular reabsorption and tubular secretion. The tubule is at all points intimately associated with the peritubular capillaries, a relationship that permits transfer of materials between the peritubular plasma and the lumen of the tubule. When the direction of transfer is from tubular lumen to peritubular-capillary plasma, the process is called *tubular reabsorption*. Movement in the opposite direction, i.e., from peritubular plasma to tubular lumen, is called *tubular secretion*. This last term must not be confused with excretion. To say that a substance has been excreted is to say that it appears in the final urine. These relationships are illustrated in Fig. 6.

The most common relationships between these basic renal processes—glomerular filtration, tubular reabsorption, and tubular secretion—are shown in Fig. 7. Plasma, containing substances X, Y, and Z, enters the glomerular capillaries. A certain quantity of protein-free plasma containing these substances is filtered into Bowman's capsule, enters the proximal tubule, and begins its flow through the rest of the tubule. The remainder of the plasma, also containing X, Y, and Z, leaves the glomerular capillaries via an efferent arteriole and enters the peritubular capillaries. The cells composing the tubular epithelium can transport X (not Y or Z) from the peritubular plasma into the tubular lumen but not in the opposite direction. By this combination of filtration and tubular secretion, all the plasma which originally entered the renal artery is cleared of substance X, which leaves the body via the urine, thus reducing the amount of X remaining in the body. If the tubule were incapable of reabsorption, the Y and Z originally filtered at the glomerulus would also leave the body via the urine, but the tubule can transport Y and Z from the tubular lumen back into the peritubular plasma. The amount of this reabsorption of Y is small, so most of the filtered material does escape from the

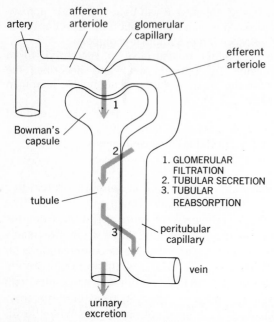

afferent
artery   arteriole   glomerular
capillary

efferent
arteriole

1

Bowman's
capsule

2

1. GLOMERULAR
   FILTRATION
2. TUBULAR SECRETION
3. TUBULAR
   REABSORPTION

tubule

3   peritubular
capillary

vein

urinary
excretion

Figure 6   The three basic components of renal function. *(From A. J. Vander et al., Human Physiology, © 1970 by McGraw-Hill, Inc. Used with permission of McGraw-Hill Book Company.)*

body. But for Z the reabsorptive mechanism is so powerful that virtually all the filtered material is reabsorbed back into the plasma, which then flows through the renal vein back into the vena cava. Therefore, no Z is lost from the body. Hence, the processes of filtration and reabsorption have canceled out each other, and the net result is as though Z had never entered the kidney at all.

The kidney works only on plasma; the erythrocytes supply oxygen to the kidney but serve no other function in urine formation. Each substance in plasma is handled in a characteristic manner by the nephron, i.e., by a particular combination of filtration, reabsorption, and secretion. (Tubular synthesis with subsequent release of the synthesized products into either the blood or the tubular lumen might well be listed as a fourth basic renal process; for example, we shall see that the tubular cells synthesize ammonia.) The critical point is that *the rates at which the relevant basic processes proceed for many of these substances are subject to physiological control.* What is the effect, for example, if the filtered mass of Y is increased or its reabsorption rate decreased? Either change causes more Y to be lost from the body via the urine. By triggering such changes in filtration or reabsorption whenever the plasma concentration of Y rises above normal, homeostatic mechanisms regulate plasma Y.

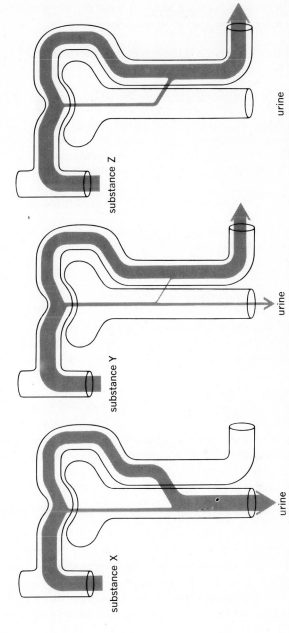

Figure 7 Renal manipulation of three substances, X, Y, and Z. X is filtered, and a fraction is then reabsorbed. Z is filtered but is completely reabsorbed. Y is filtered, and a fraction is then reabsorbed. Y is filtered and secreted but not reabsorbed. (*From A. J. Vander et al., Human Physiology, © 1970 by McGraw-Hill Book Company.*)

In summary, one can study the normal renal handling of any given substance by asking a series of questions:

1 To what degree is the substance filterable at the glomerulus?
2 Is it reabsorbed?
3 Is it secreted?
4 What are the mechanisms by which the reabsorption or secretion is achieved?
5 What factors homeostatically regulate the quantities filtered, reabsorbed, or secreted; i.e., what are the pathways by which renal excretion of the substance is altered so as to maintain stable body balance?
6 What factors other than renal disease can perturb body balance of the substance by causing the kidneys to filter, reabsorb, or secrete too much or too little of the substance?

For clinicians, of course, a seventh question must be asked: How do the various types of renal disease influence the handling of the substance and its total body balance?

GLOMERULAR FILTRATION

The capillaries of the body are freely permeable to water and to *crystalloids*, which are solutes of small molecular dimensions. They are relatively impermeable to large molecules or *colloids*, the most important of which are the plasma proteins. The glomerular capillaries behave qualitatively like any other capillary.

Composition of the Filtrate

The fluid within Bowman's capsule is essentially protein-free and contains most crystalloids in virtually the same concentrations as in the plasma.[1] These facts were established by micropuncture. Any crystalloid which is partially bound to protein has a lower concentration in Bowman's capsule than in the plasma because the protein-bound moiety will not filter. The concentration in Bowman's capsule will equal the unbound concentration in plasma.

The phrase "essentially protein-free" has been used repeatedly in referring to the glomerular filtrate. The fact is that the glomerular filtrate is not completely protein-free but does contain extremely small quantities of protein (almost entirely albumin), on the order of 50 mg/L or less. (This is less than 0.1 percent of the concentration of protein in plasma.) This protein crosses the glomerular membranes to reach Bowman's space both by

---

[1]Actually, the concentrations of charged crystalloids in Bowman's capsule are not exactly the same as in plasma because the presence of the plasma proteins causes a Donnan equilibrium to exist between these fluids, but this effect is small and may be ignored.

$^{1)}$ carriage along with the other components of the filtrate and by $^{2)}$ simple diffusion. (There is, of course, a very large diffusion gradient for protein from plasma to the fluid in Bowman's space.) In various disease states, the glomerular membranes may be altered so as to permit marked increases in the passage of protein into Bowman's space. Moreover, even in the absence of glomerular alteration, when certain proteins not normally present in the plasma appear there because of disease (for example, hemoglobin released from damaged erythrocytes and myoglobin released from damaged muscles), considerable filtration of them may occur.

Nature of the Glomerular Barrier to Macromolecules

Because, as described above, molecular size is a major factor in glomerular restriction of macromolecules, it has been convenient to view the glomerular wall as having "pores" of a certain diameter which permit complete passage of crystalloids but retard or completely impede the passage of proteins and other macromolecules (such as synthetic dextrans). On the basis of "sieving" of different-sized macromolecules, as determined experimentally, it has been possible to calculate the radius of such pores. Note that this was all based on the *functional* characteristics of the wall; are there really such anatomic pores?

It seems clear that the route through the glomerular wall taken by macromolecules, as by water and the plasma crystalloids, is completely extracellular—the fenestrae in the endothelial layer, basement membrane, slit diaphragms, and slits. Therefore, the "pores" must be sought out in this extracellular matrix. Present evidence indicates that the bulk of restriction takes place in the basement membrane and that the hydrated spaces between the elongated intertwining glycoprotein chains constituting this gellike layer are at least one component of the "pores." However, restriction by this primary filter is not absolute for most macromolecules, and some that do traverse the entire thickness of the basement membrane encounter further restriction both by the slit diaphragms and the podocyte-cell coats, which occupy much of the slits. (This is obviously a good time to reread the glomerular anatomy of Chap. 1.) The reader might well wonder what happens to macromolecules which get hung up at these sites; they are probably taken into the foot processes by endocytosis and broken down.

The discussion thus far has dealt only with steric hindrance, i.e., impairment of macromolecular movement solely because of size. Perhaps the most important recent recognition concerning glomerular selectivity is that electric charge is also a critical variable in determining penetration by proteins and other macromolecules. The molecules which constitute the extracellular matrix of the glomerular wall (the cell coats of the endothelium, the basement membrane, and the cell coats of the podocytes) are almost all polyanions. Accordingly, for any given size, negatively charged macromolecules are restricted more than neutral molecules from entering and moving through the wall, because these fixed polyanions repel them. (It is useful to imagine simply that the "pores" are lined with negative charges.) Since almost all proteins bear net negative charges, this electrical hindrance plays an important restrictive role, along with the purely steric hindrance. It is very likely that many of the diseases which cause glomeruli to be "leaky" to protein do so by eliminating many of the negative charges in the wall rather than by enlarging the "pores," as previously assumed. In leaving this topic, it must be emphasized that these negative charges act as a hindrance only to macromolecules, not to the plasma crystalloids, which are too small to be significantly influenced by any charges "lining the pores."

Forces Involved in Filtration

According to Starling's hypothesis, the *net filtration pressure* (NFP) for any capillary is the algebraic sum of the opposing hydraulic and colloid osmotic (oncotic) pressures acting across the capillary. This law also applies to the glomerular capillaries:

$$\text{NFP} = \underbrace{(P_{GC} + \pi_{BC})}_{\text{Forces inducing filtration}} - \underbrace{(P_{BC} + \pi_{GC})}_{\text{Forces opposing filtration}}$$

where P_{GC} = glomerular-capillary hydraulic pressure
π_{BC} = oncotic pressure of fluid in Bowman's capsule
P_{BC} = hydraulic pressure in Bowman's capsule
π_{GC} = oncotic pressure in glomerular-capillary plasma

Because there is virtually no protein in Bowman's capsule, π_{BC} may be taken as zero so that the equation becomes

$$\text{NFP} = P_{GC} - P_{BC} - \pi_{GC}$$

The estimated normal values of these forces in humans are given in Table 3; it must be emphasized that the relevant values (particularly that for P_{GC}) remain controversial even for experimental animals, and the values of Table 3 are only estimates based on present knowledge. Note that their magnitudes at the beginning of the glomerular capillaries differ from their magnitudes at the end of the glomerular capillaries. The changes in magnitudes are caused by two factors: (1) Capillary hydraulic pressure decreases slightly because of the resistance to flow offered by the capillaries; (2) oncotic pressure increases because, since the filtrate is essentially protein-free, the filtration process removes water but not protein

Table 3   Estimated Forces Involved in Glomerular Filtration in Humans

	mmHg	
Forces	Afferent end of glomerular capillary	Efferent end of glomerular capillary
1 Favoring filtration		
Glomerular-capillary hydraulic pressure, P_{GC}	47	45
2 Opposing filtration		
a Hydraulic pressure in Bowman's capsule, P_{BC}	10	10
b Oncotic pressure in glomerular capillary, π_{GC}	25	35
3 Net filtration pressure [(1) − (2)]	12	0

from the plasma, thereby increasing the protein concentration of the unfiltered plasma remaining in the capillaries. Normally, about 20 percent of the plasma water is filtered, accounting for the increase in oncotic pressure from 25 mmHg in the afferent end to 35 mmHg in the efferent end. The latter value for pressure is more than $25/0.8$ because the relationship between oncotic pressure and plasma protein concentration is not linear. (For complex reasons we will not describe, oncotic pressure increases more than linearly with protein concentration.)

Table 3 reveals that the net filtration pressure is quite small, 12 mmHg at the beginning of the capillary and 0 mmHg at the end. This latter number is quite significant, since it means that no filtration is occurring at all by the end of the capillary.[1] That is, the rise in oncotic pressure resulting from filtration has become high enough to completely counteract the hydraulic pressure gradient and prevent any further filtration. The figure we would like to have is the *mean net filtration pressure,* i.e., the NFP averaged over the entire capillary length. Clearly, it is somewhere between 12 and 0, but no exact number can be determined, since we do not know how soon NFP becomes 0 along the capillary. It is sufficient to recognize that the normal mean NFP is almost certainly no more than 5 to 6 mmHg. This pressure initiates urine formation by forcing an essentially protein-free filtrate of plasma through the glomerular membranes into Bowman's capsule, and thence down the tubule. In the next section we shall see that the normal rate of formation of glomerular filtrate is 125 mL/ min. That a mean net filtration pressure of only 5 to 6 mmHg or less suffices to filter this large quantity of fluid is explainable by the fact that, relative to nonrenal capillaries, the glomerular capillaries occupy a larger surface area per unit of tissue and are many times more permeable to water

[1]Whether the net filtration pressure truly reaches zero, i.e., whether filtration equilibrium occurs, is one of the major controversies concerning glomerular filtration. For the implications of this question, see the article by Blantz in Suggested Readings.

and crystalloids. It should be reemphasized that the glomerular membranes serve only as a filtration barrier and play no active, i.e., energy-requiring, role. The energy which produces glomerular filtration is the energy transmitted to the blood as hydraulic pressure when the heart contracts.

Rate of Filtration

In humans, the average volume of fluid filtered from the plasma into Bowman's capsule is 180 L/day (approximately 45 gal)! The implications of this remarkable fact are extremely important. When we recall that the average total volume of plasma in humans is approximately 3 L, it follows that the entire plasma volume is filtered by the kidneys some 60 times a day. It is, in part, this ability to process such huge volumes of plasma that enables the kidneys to excrete large quantities of waste products and to regulate the constituents of the internal environment so precisely. The second implication concerns the magnitude of the reabsorptive process. The average person excretes between 1 and 2 L of urine per day. Since 180 L of fluid are filtered, approximately 99 percent of the filtered water must have been reabsorbed into the peritubular capillaries, the remaining 1 percent escaping from the body as urinary water.

What factors directly determine the magnitude of the glomerular filtration rate? The answer is: simply the algebraic sum of the Starling forces summarized in Table 3. Accordingly, any change either in the hydraulic pressures within the glomerular capillaries or Bowman's capsule or in the oncotic pressure of the plasma can alter the net filtration pressure. For example, occlusion of the ureter will, by damming the urine, cause a rise in intratubular pressure all the way back to Bowman's capsule. The result is a decreased net filtration pressure and a reduced glomerular filtration rate. Another example: Loss of a significant quantity of protein-free extracellular fluid, such as occurs during sweating or diarrhea, increases the plasma oncotic pressure, thereby reducing net filtration pressure and glomerular filtration rate. These examples illustrate how changes either in hydraulic pressure within Bowman's capsule or in plasma oncotic pressure can alter glomerular filtration rate; changes in glomerular-capillary hydraulic pressure are also very important, and the mechanisms by which such changes are brought about are described in a subsequent chapter.

How is the rate of glomerular filtration measured (Fig. 8)? To answer this question we use another substance (let us call it W) that is freely filterable at the glomerulus but neither secreted nor reabsorbed by the tubules:

$$\frac{\text{Mass of W excreted}}{\text{Time}} = \frac{\text{mass of W filtered}}{\text{time}} \tag{1}$$

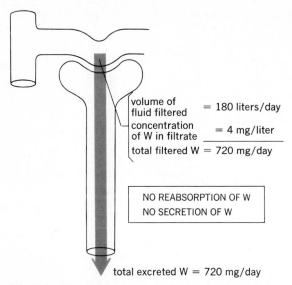

volume of
fluid filtered $= 180$ liters/day

concentration
of W in filtrate $= 4$ mg/liter

total filtered W $= 720$ mg/day

NO REABSORPTION OF W
NO SECRETION OF W

total excreted W $= 720$ mg/day

Figure 8 The measurement of glomerular filtration. W is filtered but is neither reabsorbed nor secreted. *(From A. J. Vander et al., Human Physiology, © 1970 by McGraw-Hill, Inc. Used with permission of McGraw-Hill Book Company.)*

Since the mass of any solute equals the product of solute concentration and solvent volume,

$$\frac{\text{Mass of W excreted}}{\text{Time}} = \frac{\text{urine conc of W} \times \text{urine volume}}{\text{time}} \tag{2}$$

Combining Eqs. (1) and (2):

$$U_W V = \frac{\text{mass of W filtered}}{\text{time}} \tag{3}$$

where U_W = urine concentration and V = urine volume per time.

Of course, the mass of W filtered also equals the product of the volume of plasma filtered into Bowman's capsule and the concentration of W per unit volume of filtrate. The volume of plasma filtered per unit time is, by definition, the *glomerular filtration rate* (GFR). Since W is freely filterable, the filtrate concentration of W is the same as the plasma concentration P_W. Therefore:

$$\frac{\text{Mass of W filtered}}{\text{Time}} = P_W \times \text{GFR} \tag{4}$$

Combining Eqs. (3) and (4):

$$U_W V = P_W \times \text{GFR} \tag{5}$$

Three of the variables— V, P_W, and U_W—can be measured, and we can solve for GFR:

$$\text{GFR} = \frac{U_W V}{P_W} \tag{6}$$

The validity of the above analysis depends upon the following characteristics of W:

1   Freely filterable at the glomerulus
2   Not reabsorbed
3   Not secreted
4   Not synthesized by the tubules
5   Not broken down by the tubules

A polysaccharide called *inulin* (not insulin) completely fits this description and can be used for the determination of GFR. Consider the following hypothetical situation: In order to determine your patient's GFR, you infuse inulin at a rate sufficient to maintain plasma concentration constant at 4 mg/L. Urine collected over a 2-h period has a volume of 0.2 L and an inulin concentration of 360 mg/L. What is the patient's GFR?

$$\text{GFR} = \frac{U_{In} V}{P_{In}}$$

$$\text{GFR} = \frac{360 \text{ mg/L} \times 0.2 \text{ L/2 h}}{4 \text{ mg/L}}$$

$$\text{GFR} = 18 \text{ L/2 h} = 9 \text{ L/h}$$

If any of the five criteria listed above were not valid for inulin, its use would not provide an accurate measure of GFR. For example, if inulin were secreted, which of the following statements would be true?

Calculated GFR would be higher than the true GFR.
Calculated GFR would be lower than the true GFR.

The first statement is correct because the mass of inulin excreted would represent both filtered *and* secreted inulin and, therefore, would be greater than the filtered inulin.

Once there is a means for measuring GFR, then it becomes possible to evaluate whether a substance is reabsorbed or secreted by the tubules. Thus, for any substance B which is freely filtered:

Mass of B filtered = GFR $\times P_B$

Mass of B excreted = $U_B V$

If $U_B V > (\text{GFR} \times P_B)$, then B must have been secreted

If $U_B V < (\text{GFR} \times P_B)$, then B must have been reabsorbed

Unfortunately, measuring GFR with inulin is inconvenient because inulin is not a normally occurring bodily substance and must, therefore, be administered intravenously at a continuous constant rate for several hours. Therefore, in clinical situations the indigenous substance *creatinine* is frequently used to *estimate* GFR. Creatinine is formed from muscle creatine and released into the blood at a fairly constant rate. Consequently, its blood concentration changes little during a 24-h period so that one need obtain only a single blood sample and a 24-h urine collection.

$$\text{Estimated GFR} = \frac{U_{Cr} V}{P_{Cr}}$$

This is only an estimated GFR because in humans, creatinine does not meet all five criteria; it is secreted by the tubules. It therefore overestimates the true GFR. However, the amount secreted is relatively small, and the discrepancy is not very large. In a later section we will describe how measurement of plasma creatinine alone without any urine determinations can also be used to estimate GFR more crudely. Use of urea for the same purpose will also be described.

TUBULAR REABSORPTION

Many filterable plasma components are either completely absent from the urine or present in smaller quantities than were originally filtered at the glomerulus. This fact alone is sufficient to prove that these substances undergo tubular reabsorption. An idea of the magnitude and importance of these reabsorptive mechanisms can be gained from Table 4, which summarizes data for a few plasma components, all of which are handled by filtration and reabsorption. These are typical values for a normal person on an average diet. There are at least three important conclusions to be drawn from this table: (1) The quantities of material entering the nephron via the glomerular filtrate are enormous, generally larger than their total body stores. If reabsorption of water ceased but filtration continued, the

Table 4   Average Values for Components Handled by Filtration and Reabsorption

Substance	Amount filtered per day	Amount excreted	% reabsorbed
Water, L	180	1.8	99.0
Sodium, g	630	3.2	99.5
Glucose, g	180	0	100
Urea,* g	56	28	50

*Urea handling is actually more complicated than just filtration and reabsorption. (See next chapter.)

total plasma water would be urinated within 30 min. (2) The quantities of waste products, such as urea, which are excreted in the urine are generally sizable fractions of the filtered amounts. Thus, in mammals, coupling a large glomerular filtration rate with a limited urea reabsorptive capacity permits rapid excretion of the large quantities of this substance produced constantly as a result of protein breakdown. (3) In contrast to urea and other waste products, the amount of most "useful" plasma components, e.g., water, electrolytes, and glucose, which are excreted in the urine represent quite small fractions of the filtered amounts. For this reason one often hears the generalization that the kidney performs its regulatory function by *completely* reabsorbing all of these biologically important materials and, thereby, preventing their loss from the body. This is a misleading half-truth, the refutation of which serves as an excellent opportunity for reviewing essential features of renal function and regulatory processes in general.

Let us begin by pointing out the part of the generalization that is true. Certain substances, notably glucose, are not normally excreted in the urine because the amounts filtered are completely reabsorbed by the tubules. But does such a system permit the kidneys to *regulate* the plasma concentration of glucose, i.e., *set* it at some specific concentration? The following example will point out why the answer is no. Suppose the plasma glucose concentration is 100 mg/100 mL. Since reabsorption of this carbohydrate is complete, no glucose is lost from the body via the urine, and the plasma concentration remains at 100 mg/100 mL. If, instead of 100 mg/100 mL, we set our hypothetical plasma glucose concentration at 60 mg/100 mL, the analysis does not change; no glucose is lost in the urine and the plasma glucose stays at 60 mg/100 mL. Obviously, the kidney is merely maintaining whatever plasma glucose concentration happens to exist and is not involved in the regulatory mechanisms by which the original setting of the plasma glucose was accomplished. It is not the kidney but primarily the liver and the endocrine system which set and regulate the plasma glucose concentration.[1] For comparison, consider what happens when a person drinks a lot of water: Within 1 to 2 h all the excess has been excreted in the urine, chiefly, as we shall see, as the result of decreased renal tubular reabsorption of water. In this example the kidney is the effector organ of a reflex which maintains plasma water concentration within very narrow limits. The critical point is that for many "useful" plasma components, particularly the inorganic ions and water, the kidney does *not completely* reabsorb the total amounts filtered. The rates at which these substances are reabsorbed (and, therefore, the rates at which they are excreted) are constantly subject to physiological control. This ability to vary the reabsorption rates of water, sodium, calcium, phosphate, and many other substances (and to vary the secretion rates of still others) is really the essence of the kidney's ability to regulate the internal environment.

A bewildering variety of ions and molecules is found in the plasma and, therefore, in the glomerular filtrate, and most are reabsorbed to varying extents. It is essential to realize that tubular reabsorption is a qualitatively different process from glomerular filtration. The latter occurs by bulk flow, in which water and all dissolved free (non-protein-bound) crystalloids move together; this bulk flow occurs both because the appropriate net filtration pressure exists to drive it and because the glomerular wall has "pores" large enough to permit fluid flow. In contrast, there is relatively little bulk flow across the tubular-epithelial cells from lumen to interstitium because neither of these conditions is met; there are little, if any, hydraulic and oncotic pressure gradients, and the tubular epithelium is relatively "nonporous." (Recall that tubular-epithelial cells are joined together by tight junctions.) It must be emphasized that we are speaking here only of the relative lack of bulk flow from tubular lumen to interstitium; as will be discussed in Chap. 6, there is considerable bulk flow from interstitial fluid into peritubular capillaries, and this constitutes one of the ways (diffusion being the other) for a reabsorbed substance, having made it from tubular lumen to interstitial fluid, to complete its journey by gaining entry to the peritubular capillaries.

Given that bulk flow is not an important mechanism for transport of substances across the tubular-epithelial cells, it follows that tubular reabsorption of various substances is not by mass movement but rather by more or less discrete transport processes. The phrase "more or less discrete" denotes several important facts: (1) The reabsorption of different

---

[1]Time and research give the lie to all generalizations. It is now known that the renal tubular cells actually *synthesize* glucose and release it into the blood during a prolonged fast. In this manner the kidneys do help set the plasma glucose concentration during prolonged fasting. This in no way detracts from the discussion above, which describes how glucose *reabsorption* does *not* contribute to the setting.

substances may be linked (for example, the reabsorption of many amino acids, glucose, and other solutes is linked to that of sodium); (2) a single reabsorptive system may be capable of transporting several distinct, but structurally similar, substances (for example, at least four of the simple carbohydrates are reabsorbed by a single system).

What are these transport mechanisms involved in tubular reabsorption? They are basically the same mechanisms involved in membrane transport anywhere in the body, and any discussion of transport is complicated by the problem of terminology. The traditional division between "active" and "passive" transport breaks down rather quickly when one focuses on mechanisms, and the following classification is proving more meaningful at present.

Classification of Transport Mechanisms

Simple Diffusion   This process is due to random molecular motion and requires the presence of an electrochemical gradient for net movement to occur; i.e., net diffusion is always "downhill." Because simple diffusion proceeds mainly through the lipid matrix of the membrane, lipid solubility is a major determinant of any substance's diffusibility; only very small polar substances penetrate to any great extent by simple diffusion, presumably because they move through water-filled spaces trapped in the lipid matrix or water-filled "pores" created by the arrangement of the membrane's proteins. In contrast to the next four transport processes to be listed, simple diffusion involves no specific interaction between the moving molecule and the proteins of the membrane.

Simple Facilitated Diffusion   This process, like simple diffusion, can produce net movement of a substance only down its electrochemical gradient (thus, the term "diffusion"). However, unlike simple diffusion, the transport is dependent upon interaction of the substance with specific membrane proteins, which "facilitate" its movement; therefore, the rate of movement is much higher than would be expected by simple diffusion (but, to reiterate, net movement is still downhill). This is an important mechanism for accelerating the movement of non-lipid-soluble molecules, and the membrane proteins involved are frequently termed "carriers." The initial event in facilitated diffusion is the binding of the molecule to be transported to the carrier, but the next events which actually lead to facilitation of the molecule's translocation across the membrane remain unknown. Because of the interaction with membrane proteins, facilitated diffusion manifests the characteristics of specificity, saturability, and competition; none of these characteristics is exhibited by simple diffusion.

Coupled Facilitated Diffusion of Two or More Substances   In this process, two (or sometimes more) substances interact simultaneously with the same specific membrane proteins (carriers), and both are translocated across the membrane by facilitated diffusion. Such co-transport manifests specificity, saturability, and competition, just as does simple facilitated diffusion. Why, then, treat this as a separate category? Because the result of coupled facilitated diffusion may differ from that of simple facilitated diffusion in a crucial way: There can occur net movement of one of the co-transported substances *uphill,* i.e., against its electrochemical gradient. Thermodynamic considerations demand that net uphill transport utilize energy, so that we must ask what is the source of energy in such a process. The answer is the energy liberated by the simultaneous downhill diffusion of the other co-transported substance. In other words, as one of the substances moves with its electrochemical gradient, the energy released somehow is able to drive the other substance uphill against its electrochemical gradient; we simply do not have any simple model to explain how this actually operates on a molecular level. Sodium is frequently the substance moving downhill in coupled facilitated diffusion systems, and the co-transported substance being simultaneously moved uphill is said to undergo *secondary active transport.* (The derivation of this term will be clarified in a subsequent section.)

Primary (Traditional) Active Transport   In this process, the transported molecule also interacts with membrane proteins (carriers) and may exhibit specificity, saturability, and competition. Its hallmark is net uphill transport, with the energy for this "active" transport coming *directly* from the splitting of ATP or from some other source of chemical energy. (Contrast this to the concentration-gradient source of energy utilized by "secondary active transport" systems, as described above.) Indeed, the term "primary" specifically denotes that chemical energy is the direct source of the energy for the process, and, in some cases, membrane-bound ATPase not only splits the ATP to provide energy but is a component of the actual carrier mechanism.

Endocytosis   This process is characterized by the invagination of a portion of the plasma membrane until it becomes completely pinched off and exists as an isolated intracellular membrane-bound vesicle filled with the extracellular fluid it imbibed during its formation. This process offers an important mechanism for the uptake of macromolecules, which may trigger off the entire process by binding to specific membrane proteins. Endocytosis, of course, requires energy, and its source is the splitting of ATP. (Thus, endocytosis is a form of primary active transport.)

Transport Mechanisms in Reabsorption

We began this discussion of tubular reabsorptive mechanisms with the statement that they are simply the basic mechanisms for transport across any cell membranes, but we must now face the added complexity that arises when one deals with an epithelial layer, such as the renal tubule (or gastrointestinal epithelium, gallbladder epithelium, etc.), rather than the plasma membrane of a single nonepithelial cell (a muscle cell or erythrocyte, for example). The problem is quite straightforward: Except for the few substances which are reabsorbed by simple diffusion across the tight junctions *between* cells, all other reabsorbed substances must cross *two* membranes in their journey from tubular lumen to interstitial fluid—the *luminal membrane* (separating the luminal fluid from the cell cytoplasm) and the *basolateral membrane* (separating the cytoplasm from the interstitial fluid). (The boundary between the luminal and basolateral membranes is the tight junction.) Accordingly, in order to fully characterize the overall transport of a substance across the epithelium, one must know what transport characteristics exist for each membrane.

Let us take sodium reabsorption as an example (Fig. 9). Sodium ions move across the luminal membrane into cell cytoplasm mainly by simple facilitated diffusion. They are then actively transported across the basolateral membrane into the interstitial fluid. This latter "pump" is a primary active process which involves Na-K–dependent ATPase found only in the basolateral membranes. Finally, the sodium ions, along with water, move into the peritubular capillaries by bulk flow. (Bulk flow or simple diffusion into the peritubular capillaries is the final step in the reabsorption of all substances.) Thus, the unidirectional reabsorptive movement of sodium is made possible by the asymmetry of the luminal and basolateral membrane transport processes. What may not be apparent from this brief description is the fact that the luminal and basolateral events do not occur in isolation from each other. This becomes evident as soon as one recognizes that the continued net movement of sodium across the luminal membrane (being a simple facilitated diffusion process) depends completely upon the maintenance of a favorable electrochemical gradient—cytoplasmic [Na] < luminal [Na] and electric potential oriented so that the cell interior is negative relative to the lumen. The crucial point is that the basolateral pump creates this electrochemical gradient by keeping the cytoplasmic [Na] low and the cell interior negatively charged. (The exact role of the sodium pump in the creation of intracellular negativity is complex and need not be dealt with here.)

Let us take another example, the reabsorption of glucose (Fig. 10). Glucose moves from the lumen across the luminal membrane into the cell cytoplasm by coupled facilitated diffusion with sodium. (This carrier is quite distinct from the simple facilitated diffusion carrier used by most

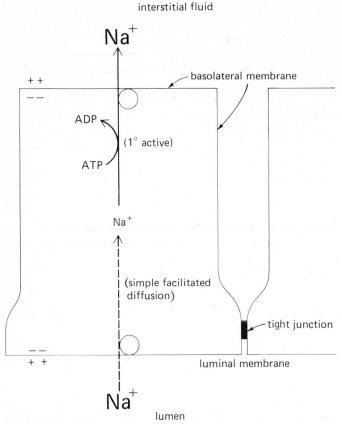

interstitial fluid

Figure 9 Reabsorption of sodium. Net facilitated diffusion into the cell is made possible by the low cytoplasmic [Na] and the potential difference, both ultimately the result of the basolateral primary active "pump."

sodium ions; i.e., sodium moves into the cell by a variety of facilitated diffusion pathways.) Note that the glucose uptake is an example of uphill transport characteristic of coupled facilitated diffusion systems—the energy utilized to drive uphill movement of glucose is derived from the simultaneous downhill movement of sodium. So efficient is this uphill movement that the lumen can be virtually cleared of glucose. After entry into the cell, the glucose then exits across the basolateral membrane by simple facilitated diffusion, this downhill movement being driven by the high glucose concentration achieved in the cell by the action of the luminal transport process. A critical point, easy to miss, is that the entire overall process of glucose reabsorption depends ultimately upon the primary active sodium pump in the basolateral membrane! Only because

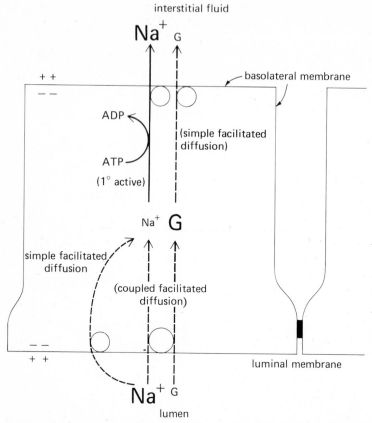

Figure 10 "Secondary active reabsorption" of glucose. Follow this figure by beginning with the primary active Na pump in the basolateral membrane. Then you will see
how the low intracellular [Na] and intracellular negativity permit the net downhill entry
of Na across the luminal membrane, which, in turn, provides the energy for simultaneous uphill glucose movement across this membrane. Luminal [glucose] is shown falling toward zero as it is reabsorbed.

of this pump is the electrochemical gradient maintained for net sodium diffusion across the luminal membrane, and it is this downhill process that
provides the energy for the simultaneous uphill movement of the glucose.
Now the reader should be able to understand why glucose reabsorption is
termed secondary active transport—it is itself uphill ("active") but is
"secondary" to (dependent upon) "primary" active sodium transport.
Instead of glucose, we could have used amino acids, phosphate, or a variety of organic substances as our example, for they, too, undergo secondary active reabsorption by being co-transported with sodium in precisely
the same manner.

Despite the breakdown of the traditional categorization of transport processes as "active" or "passive," renal physiologists still find it helpful to use these terms to characterize the overall reabsorptive process for any given substance. In such usage, "active" simply is a shorthand way of stating that at least one of the two membrane crossings is achieved by a primary or secondary active process, i.e., that uphill transport against the substance's electrochemical gradient has occurred somewhere between lumen and interstitial fluid. Thus, we say that glucose undergoes active reabsorption.

Transport Maximum

Many of the active reabsorptive systems in the renal tubule can transport only limited amounts of material per unit time, primarily because the membrane proteins somehow responsible for the transport become saturated. The classical example is the transport process for glucose in the proximal tubule. As we have seen, normal persons do not excrete glucose in their urine because tubular reabsorption is complete. But it is possible to produce urinary excretion of glucose in a completely normal person merely by administering large quantities of glucose directly into a vein (Table 5).

Note that even after the plasma glucose concentration has doubled, the urine is still glucose-free, indicating that the _maximal tubular transport capacity_ (T_m) for reabsorbing glucose has not yet been reached. But as the plasma glucose and the filtered load continue to rise, glucose finally appears in the urine. From this point on, any further increase in plasma glucose is accompanied by a proportionate increase in excreted glucose because the T_m, which equals 375 mg/min, has now been reached. The tubules are now reabsorbing all the glucose they can, and any amount filtered in excess of this quantity cannot be reabsorbed and appears in the urine. This is precisely what occurs in the patient with diabetes mellitus. Because of a deficiency in pancreatic production of insulin, the patient's

Table 5 Experimental Data Obtained for Calculation of Glucose T_m

Time, min	GFR, mL/min	P_G, mg/mL	Filtered glucose (GFR $\times$ P_G), mg/min	Excreted glucose $(U_G V)$, mg/min	Reabsorbed glucose (filtered−excreted), mg/min
0	125	1.0	125	0	125
Begin glucose infusion					
26–40	125	2.0	250	0	250
100–110	125	4.0	500	125	375
130–140	125	5.0	625	250	375

plasma glucose may rise to extremely high values. The filtered load of glucose becomes great enough to exceed the T_m, and glucose appears in the urine. There is nothing wrong with the tubular transport mechanism for glucose. It is simply unable to reabsorb the huge filtered load.

To add one more level of complexity, let us return to the experiment in which glucose was infused. Additional data were obtained for minutes 60 to 100 but were not shown in Table 5. They are as follows:

Time, min	GFR, mL/min	P_G, mg/mL	Filtered glucose, mg/min	Excreted glucose, mg/min	Reabsorbed glucose, mg/min
60–80	125	2.8	350	20	330
80–100	125	3.5	436	76	360

Now we see that glucose began to be excreted in the urine *before* the true T_m of 375 mg/min was reached. There are several reasons for this so-called splay: (1) A carrier-mediated mechanism shows kinetics analogous to those of enzyme systems so that maximal activity is substrate-dependent (in this case, glucose-dependent); i.e., the pump may not work at its absolute maximal rate until the luminal glucose concentration is too high to permit all of it to be "captured" by the pump. (2) Not all nephrons have the same T_m for glucose so that some may be spilling glucose at a time when others have not yet reached their T_m's. This last point is extremely important, for we too often fall into the habit of viewing the kidneys as one large nephron. The fact is that there are really over 2 million nephrons in the kidneys, and they are not completely identical in functional characteristics.

Except for our experimental subject receiving intravenous glucose, the plasma glucose in normal persons never becomes high enough to cause urinary excretion of glucose because the reabsorptive capacity for glucose is much greater than necessary for normal filtered loads. However, for certain other substances, e.g., phosphate, the reabsorptive T_m is very close to the normal filtered load. The adaptive value inherent in such a relationship should be readily apparent from the following example: On a normal person the following data are obtained:

$$\text{Ingested PO}_4 = 20 \text{ mmol/day}$$
$$\text{GFR} = 180 \text{ L/day}$$
$$\text{Plasma PO}_4 \text{ conc} = 1 \text{ mmol/L}^1$$
$$\text{Filtered PO}_4 = 1 \times 180 = 180 \text{ mmol/day}$$
$$T_m \text{ for PO}_4 = 160 \text{ mmol/day}$$
$$\text{Excreted PO}_4 = 180 - 160 = 20 \text{ mmol/day}$$

---

[1] A small fraction of plasma phosphate is bound to protein. The value given here is the ultrafilterable concentration.

Under these conditions the normal person remains in perfect phosphate balance since what is eaten is excreted and plasma phosphate concentration therefore remains constant at 1 mmol/L. If the next day the same person eats an unusually large quantity of phosphate and raises the plasma phosphate concentration to 1.1 mmol/L, the data are

$$GFR = 180 \text{ L/day}$$
$$\text{Filtered PO}_4 = 1.1 \times 180 = 198 \text{ mmol/day}$$
$$T_m \text{ for PO}_4 = 160 \text{ mmol/day}$$
$$\text{Excreted PO}_4 = 198 - 160 = 38 \text{ mmol/day}$$

The very slight increase in plasma phosphate has resulted in a large increase in excreted phosphate and has eliminated the excess phosphate ingested. By this mechanism, depending on neither hormones nor nerves, the kidney can exert control over plasma phosphate concentration. (We shall see that, in addition to this simplest of systems, more complex systems involving hormonal components also exist for the regulation of phosphate.)

TUBULAR SECRETION

Tubular secretory processes, which transport substances across the tubular epithelium into the lumen, i.e., in the direction opposite to tubular reabsorption, constitute a second pathway into the tubule, the first pathway being glomerular filtration. We need say little about the types of transport mechanisms which achieve tubular secretion because they are the same as those previously described for tubular reabsorption, i.e., simple diffusion, simple and coupled facilitated diffusion, and primary active transport. (Endocytosis is not an important mechanism for tubular secretion.)

The overall secretory process for any given substance begins with its simple diffusion out of the peritubular capillaries into the interstitial fluid, from which it makes its way into the lumen by crossing either the tight junctions (in some cases of simple diffusion) or, in turn, the basolateral and luminal membranes of the cell. In the latter cases, the net unidirectional movement usually results from differences in the characteristics of the two membranes. For example (Fig. 11), the secreted substance might be pumped across the basolateral membrane by a primary active process, and the resulting high intracellular concentration could then drive movement across the luminal membrane by diffusion (either simple or facilitated). Of course, other possible combinations could achieve the same final result, i.e., net movement into the tubular lumen. For the great majority of secreted substances, we are not yet completely certain as to just which combinations do exist. As is true for tubular reabsorption, the overall process of tubular secretion can be categorized as active or pas-

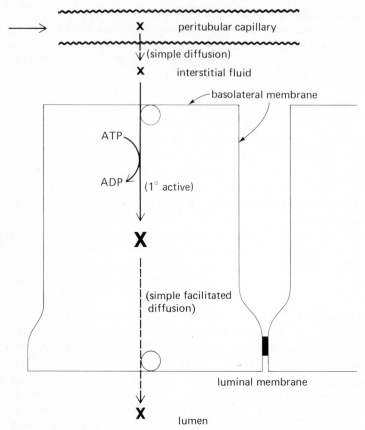

Figure 11 Secretory pathway for hypothetical substance X.

sive depending upon whether an uphill process occurs at one or both membranes.

Among the most important secretory processes are those for hydrogen ion and potassium, and these will be discussed in detail later. There exist in the proximal tubule several low-specificity secretory systems for organic molecules. (See Chap. 3.) These are analogous to the proximal reabsorptive mechanisms described above for glucose and phosphate in that they are active, are T_m-limited, manifest competition, and can be inhibited by various drugs. One transport mechanism secretes a variety of normally occurring foreign organic anions, including para-aminohippurate and penicillin. A second system secretes many organic bases, both endogenous and foreign. There may be more. The fact that these secretory mechanisms are relatively nondiscriminating and can transport foreign substances makes them important for the elimination from the body of drugs and other foreign environmental chemicals. Here, the liver's metabolic transformations are frequently important. In the liver, many foreign (and endogenous) substances are conjugated with glucuronic acid or sulfate; these two categories of molecules are actively transported by the organic anion secretory pathway.

BIDIRECTIONAL TRANSPORT

In the preceding sections, the adjective "net" was frequently used in reference to tubular reabsorption or secretion and was always implicit even when absent. The fact is that only rarely, if ever, does any transported substance manifest purely unidirectional flux across the tubule totally unopposed by a flux in the other direction. One reason for this is that the epithelium is not completely impermeable to crystalloids so that bidirectional diffusion is always occurring even in the absence of diffusion gradients.

Another reason is apparent from reconsideration of the example illustrated in Fig. 11. Note that, because of the primary active transport process in the basolateral membrane, the overall secretory process achieves a concentration gradient between lumen and interstitial fluid. This gradient, of course, favors a net movement by simple diffusion in the reabsorptive direction so that if the tight junctions or cell membranes themselves are at all permeable to substance X, such movement will occur. This is an example of a so-called pump-leak system, in which the active "pump" creates a diffusion gradient which opposes its own action by favoring back-diffusion. Since this back-diffusion occurs solely as an indirect result of the pump's activity and since the net flux will, therefore, always be in the direction of the pump, we do not usually dignify the back-diffusion with the terms reabsorption or secretion. In other words, in reference to Fig. 11, we say simply that X is handled by secretion (and do not call the passive back-flux "reabsorption"). To take the sodium pattern of Fig. 9 as another example, we say simply that sodium is reabsorbed (and do not assign the term "secretion" to the passive back flux into the lumen secondary to the concentration gradient created by the sodium pump).

A quite different situation exists when a nephron segment contains distinct opposing pathways or "reversible pumps" for a single substance. This may seem strange, but such systems do exist, and the nephron segment may, therefore, manifest net secretion or net reabsorption depending upon the physiological circumstances.

Finally, for many substances, a given nephron segment may always manifest only reabsorption or only secretion, but other nephron segments may do just the opposite. For example, a substance may be secreted into the proximal tubule but reabsorbed from the distal tubule; in such cases, the relative magnitudes of the opposing processes in the different nephron segments determine whether the overall tubular effect will be reabsorption or secretion.

METABOLISM BY THE TUBULES

Although renal physiologists have traditionally listed glomerular filtration, tubular reabsorption, and tubular secretion as the three basic renal processes, a fourth fate is also of considerable importance for many substances—metabolism by the tubular cells. For example, the cells may extract organic nutrients from the peritubular capillaries but rather than secreting them into the lumen, the cells may metabolize them as dictated by the cells' own nutrient requirements. In so doing, the renal cells are behaving no differently than any other cells in the body.

In contrast, other metabolic transformations performed by the kidney are not directed toward its own nutritional requirements but rather toward altering the composition of the urine. The most important of these is the synthesis of ammonia from glutamine, as described in Chap. 9.

Study questions: **3 to 7**

Chapter 3

Renal Handling of Organic Substances

OBJECTIVES

Student understands the renal handling of certain organic substances.
1 States the major characteristics of the proximal-tubular systems for reabsorption of organic nutrients
2 Describes the renal handling of protein; calculates the mass filtered and reabsorbed
3 Describes the renal handling of urea
4 Describes the renal handling of uric acid
5 Describes the renal handling of creatinine
6 Describes, in general terms, the renal handling of weak acids and bases, including the contributions of active secretion and passive movements secondary to water reabsorption or pH changes; given any change in luminal pH, predicts the change in net transtubular movement.

All subsequent chapters of this book will deal almost exclusively with the renal handling of inorganic substances, since regulation of their excretion constitutes the kidneys' major physiological role. However, as pointed out in Chap. 1, another major renal function is the excretion of organic waste products, foreign chemicals, and their metabolites. Moreover, reabsorptive processes must exist to prevent massive excretion of filtered organic nutrients. An analysis of the renal transport pathways for all these organic substances is well beyond the scope of this book, but this chapter briefly describes certain of them, the major goal being to summarize and further illustrate the basic principles described in the previous chapter.

GLUCOSE, AMINO ACIDS, ET AL.; PROXIMAL REABSORPTION OF ORGANIC NUTRIENTS

The proximal tubule is the major site of reabsorption of the large quantities of organic nutrients filtered each day by the glomeruli. These include glucose, amino acids, several Krebs cycle intermediates, certain water-soluble vitamins, lactate, acetoacetate, β-hydroxybutyrate, and still others. The characteristics of glucose reabsorption described in examples used earlier in Chap. 2 are typical of the transport processes for most (but not all) of them:

    1   They are active in that they can reabsorb their respective solutes against electrochemical gradients, often reducing the intraluminal concentration virtually to zero.

    2   Co-transport with sodium is involved; i.e., the uphill steps are "secondary active" processes.

    3   They manifest T_m's which are usually well above the amounts *normally* filtered; accordingly, the kidneys protect against loss of the substances but do not help set their plasma concentrations. However, as we saw for glucose in diabetic persons, under abnormal conditions, the plasma concentration of any of these substances may become so increased as to cause the reabsorptive T_m for it to be exceeded and large quantities to be lost in the urine. Good examples are acetoacetate and β-hydroxybutyrate in patients with severe uncontrolled diabetes.

    4   They manifest specificity. This means that there are a large number of different "carriers" (i.e., membrane proteins with which the different solute types interact). But there is by no means a one-to-one correspondence, since two or more closely related substances may utilize the same carrier. For example, the amino acid reabsorptive mechanisms are quite distinct from those for glucose (and other monosaccharides), but there are not 20 separate processes (one for each amino acid); rather there is one for arginine, lysine, ornithine, and cystine; another for glutamate and aspartate; and so on. The existence of shared pathways allows for competition among those substances utilizing any given pathway; for example, the administration of large quantities of ornithine partially blocks the reabsorption of the other three amino acids which share its pathway. (This is, of course, explainable on the basis of competition for the common carrier's binding sites.)

    5   They are inhibitable by a variety of drugs and diseases. There are persons with genetic defects manifested as a deficit in one or more of these proximal reabsorptive systems (so-called inborn errors of transport). In some cases, the deficit may be highly specific (involving only one amino acid, for example), whereas in others, multiple systems may be involved (glucose and many amino acids, for example). This range of defects is also seen when the deficit is due to an external agent rather than to a genetic abnormality.

PROTEIN

The proximal tubule is also the major site for protein reabsorption, but it is listed separately here to emphasize its importance and the fact that its reabsorptive pathway is quite different from those for the substances listed in the preceding section. As mentioned above, there is a very small amount of protein in the glomerular filtrate. The exact normal concentration is unknown but is now thought to approximate 20 mg/L, about 0.04 percent of plasma albumin concentration. Yet this is *not* negligible because of the huge volume of fluid filtered per day.

$$
\begin{aligned}
\text{Total filtered protein} &= \text{GFR} \times \text{filtrate conc of protein} \\
&= 180 \text{ L/day} \times 20 \text{ mg/L} \\
&= 3.6 \text{ g/day}
\end{aligned}
$$

If none of this protein were reabsorbed, the entire 3.6 g would be lost in the urine. In fact, virtually all of the filtered protein is reabsorbed so that the excretion of protein in the urine is normally only 100 mg/day. The mechanism by which protein is reabsorbed is easily saturated, so any large increase in filtered protein resulting from increased glomerular permeability can cause the excretion of large quantities of protein. For example, suppose that disease causes the glomeruli to allow 1 percent of the plasma albumin to be filtered:

$$
\begin{aligned}
\text{Filtered protein} &= \text{GFR} \times (50 \text{ g/L}) (0.01) \\
&= 180 \text{ L/day} \times 0.5 \text{ g/L} \\
&= 90 \text{ g/day}
\end{aligned}
$$

This is far greater than the protein T_m, and large quantities of protein would be lost in the urine.

The initial step in protein reabsorption is endocytosis at the luminal membrane. This energy-requiring process is triggered by the binding of filtered protein molecules to specific sites on the luminal membranes; therefore, the rate of endocytosis is increased in proportion to the concentration of protein in the glomerular filtrate until a maximal rate of vesicle formation (and, thus, the T_m for protein reabsorption) is reached. The pinched-off intracellular vesicles resulting from endocytosis merge with lysosomes, whose enzymes degrade the protein to low-molecular-weight fragments. These end products are then released across the basolateral membrane into the interstitial fluid, from which they gain entry to the peritubular capillaries. It should be evident from this description that the term *reabsorption,* in reference to protein handling, is a bit unusual, since the intact protein molecules themselves are not actually being moved from lumen to interstitial fluid. (There may be a small number which actually do, since a few intact endocytotic vesicles move through the cell cytoplasm and empty their proteins by exocytosis into the interstitial fluid.) Nevertheless, the important point is that the filtered protein is not excreted in the urine and is, in this sense, reabsorbed.

UREA

Just as glucose provides an excellent example of an actively transported solute, urea (the primary end product of protein catabolism) provides an example of transport by simple diffusion. Urea is a highly diffusible substance so that net movement across most biological membranes requires only the creation of a diffusion gradient for it. Such gradients exist within the kidneys, as the following analysis shows.

Since urea is freely filtered at the glomerulus, its concentration in Bowman's capsule is identical to its concentration in peritubular-capillary plasma. Then, as the fluid flows along the proximal tubule, water reabsorption occurs, increasing the concentration of any intratubular solute not being reabsorbed at the same rate as the water. As a result, the concentration of urea in the tubular lumen becomes greater than the concen-

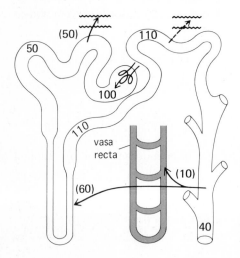

Figure 12 Renal handling of urea. The numbers in parentheses denote the percentages of filtered urea present at various sites along the tubule. *(Redrawn from H. Valtin, Renal Function: Mechanisms Preserving Fluid and Solute Balance in Health, Little, Brown, Boston, 1973.)*

tration of urea in the peritubular plasma. Accordingly, urea is able to diffuse passively down this concentration gradient from tubular lumen to interstitial fluid, and then into peritubular capillaries. Urea reabsorption is, thus, a passive process and completely dependent upon water reabsorption, which establishes the diffusion gradient.

This passive reabsorption of urea is not limited to the proximal tubule but also occurs in other nephron segments as water continues to be reabsorbed. However, beyond the proximal tubule, the story becomes much more complicated. Let us pick up the fluid at the end of the proximal tubule, at which point approximately 50 percent of the urea has been reabsorbed,[1] and follow it the rest of the way, using Fig. 12 as reference.

What happens in the loop of Henle? One might logically have predicted that more urea would be reabsorbed along with the water reabsorbed from the loop (water reabsorption by the loop is described in Chap. 6), but such turns out not to be the case. By the beginning of the distal tubule, there is actually twice as much urea in the tubular fluid as originally left the proximal tubule (i.e., about the same amount as originally filtered)! Thus, *secretion* of urea into the loop of Henle has occurred. However, the source of this secreted urea is *not* peritubular plasma (the usual source of secreted solutes) and is best ignored for the present until we complete the tubular fluid's journey through the nephron.

Some of this enlarged amount of urea is reabsorbed (again by simple diffusion down its concentration gradient) in the distal tubule, but not much because the distal tubule is not very permeable to it. Therefore, most of the urea which entered the distal tubule from the loop drains into the collecting ducts. There, particularly in the segment of collecting duct in the inner medulla, passive urea reabsorption once again becomes quite large both because of a high tubular permeability to urea and because of the extensive water reabsorption there. The urea which escapes reabsorption by the collecting ducts amounts to approximately 40 percent of the

---

[1]This seems a good place to describe how such information is obtained using micropuncture. A sample of fluid is collected from the end of the proximal tubule, and its concentrations of inulin and urea are measured and compared to those of arterial plasma. The percent of filtered urea remaining at the end of the proximal tubule is given by the ratio:

$$\frac{\dfrac{\text{Tubular fluid}_{\text{urea}}}{\text{Plasma}_{\text{urea}}}}{\dfrac{\text{Tubular fluid}_{\text{In}}}{\text{Plasma}_{\text{In}}}} \times 100$$

Any value greater than 100 percent means, of course, that secretion has occurred, less than 100 percent signifies reabsorption. A careful look at this equation should reveal that it is really the clearance concept all over again. To determine what the loop has done, a sample is collected from the early distal and the "double ratio" compared to that for the late proximal. This early distal sample can then be compared to a late distal one to evaluate the contribution of the distal tubule.

amount originally filtered, and this is the urea excreted into the final urine. Thus, the *overall net* renal tubular handling of urea is the reabsorption of approximately 60 percent.

Now we can back up and point out the source of the urea which entered the loop of Henle by secretion—it is most of the urea which is reabsorbed by the collecting ducts! The key point, illustrated in Fig. 12, is that the medullary collecting ducts and the thin limbs of the loops of Henle are parallel to each other and share the same interstitial fluid; therefore, as urea diffuses out of the collecting ducts into the interstitial fluid, the urea concentration of this fluid is raised, thereby creating a gradient for net diffusion of urea into the thin limbs. This movement is restricted mainly to the thin ascending limb, which has a much greater permeability to urea than does the thin descending limb.

Thus, most of the urea which diffuses *out of* the collecting ducts (reabsorption) diffuses *into* the loops (secretion) and once more flows through the distal nephron only to suffer the same fate again in the collecting ducts. In other words, a large quantity of urea is simply recycled between these segments of the nephron. Not all the urea which diffuses out of the collecting ducts is recycled in this manner, since some enters the medullary capillaries and is carried out of the kidneys.

In summary (Fig. 12), the renal handling of filtered urea is by simple diffusion. Approximately 50 percent is reabsorbed into the blood across the proximal tubule. The remaining 50 percent undergoes a recycling sequence beyond the proximal tubule characterized by reabsorption out of the collecting ducts followed by secretion into the loop of Henle. Approximately 10 percent of the filtered urea escapes this recycling and makes it into the capillaries and back into the systemic circulation. The net result is that approximately 60 percent (50 percent by the proximal and 10 percent by the rest of the nephron) of the filtered urea is truly (in the sense of "irrevocably") reabsorbed. This figure of 60 percent reabsorbed applies to situations in which the urine flow is relatively low (i.e., water reabsorption high). Only about 40 percent of the filtered urea is reabsorbed when the urine flow is high (i.e., water reabsorption low). This is because the diffusion gradient for urea reabsorption is created by water reabsorption, and the less the latter, the less will be the former.

To reiterate, the net reabsorption of filtered urea ranges between 40 and 60 percent. A crucial fact is that this same range applies regardless of how high the plasma urea concentration may be. Thus, urea reabsorption manifests no true T_m, in absolute terms, because it is governed by simple diffusion gradients and requires no interaction with membrane binding sites. The clinical implications of this absence of a T_m and the relatively small changes in the percentage reabsorbed will be described in the next chapter.

URIC ACID

Uric acid excretion in a normal person is approximately 700 mg/day; its concentration in plasma equals 5 mg/100 mL. How is uric acid handled by the kidney? First, we ascertain that uric acid is not protein-bound and that it is freely filterable. Therefore, we can now measure the quantity of uric acid filtered per unit time.

$$\text{Filtered uric acid} = \text{GFR} \times P_{\text{uric acid}}$$
$$= 180 \text{ L/day} \times 50 \text{ mg/L}$$
$$= 9000 \text{ mg/day}$$

We can now say for certain that uric acid is reabsorbed by the tubules because the mass excreted per unit time is less than the mass filtered. Does this prove that uric acid is not secreted by the tubules? The answer is *no*. Secretion might be occurring at a much lower rate than reabsorption, which would, therefore, mask it. Indeed, such is the case with uric acid. Thus, we have a substance which is both reabsorbed and secreted, both processes being carrier-mediated and occurring mainly in the proximal tubule.

As might be imagined, the existence of bidirectional carrier-mediated transport processes has greatly complicated attempts to understand the mechanisms and controls of uric acid excretion. For example, many persons have elevated plasma concentrations of uric acid because they excrete less of this substance at any given plasma concentration than do normal persons. Is this because of defective secretion or overzealous reabsorption? Similarly, it has been difficult to nail down the ways in which various drugs given to such persons to increase uric acid excretion work; do they enhance secretion or block reabsorption?

CREATININE

This end product of creatine metabolism is completely filterable at the glomerulus and does not undergo tubular reabsorption. A small amount is secreted, mainly by the proximal tubules, so that its total excretion reflects this secreted moiety along with the much larger amount filtered. It is mentioned here because of its great importance in the chemical evaluation of renal function. (See next chapter.)

WEAK ORGANIC ACIDS AND BASES

The most striking fact concerning the overall renal handling of weak organic acids and bases, some indigenous to the body but many more foreign (drugs, food additives, environmental pollutants, etc.), is that either net secretion or net reabsorption may occur, depending upon several conditions, the most important being the pH of the urine. To be specific, many weak acids undergo net tubular secretion when the urine is highly alkaline but net tubular reabsorption when it is acidic. The opposite pattern is seen for many weak organic bases.

To understand what accounts for this pH dependency, one must realize that the renal tubular epithelium, like other biological membranes, is mainly a lipid barrier; accordingly, highly lipid-soluble substances can penetrate it fairly readily by simple diffusion. Recall that one of the major determinants of lipid solubility is the polarity of a molecule; the more polar, the less lipid-soluble. Now, a weak acid exists as a polar ion in alkaline solution and as a nonpolar molecule in acid solution (the exact pH dependency of this reaction depends, of course, on the pK of the molecules in question):

$$A^- + H^+ \rightleftharpoons AH$$

For weak bases, the ionic form is favored in acid solutions.

$$B + H^+ \rightleftharpoons BH^+$$

Accordingly, the diffusible form of weak acids is generated in acidic fluid, whereas the diffusible form of weak bases is generated in alkaline fluid.

Let us now apply these principles using aspirin as an example:

$$ASA^- \quad + H^+ \rightleftharpoons \quad ASA\text{-}H$$
$$\text{(acetylsalicylate)} \qquad \text{(acetylsalicylic acid)}$$

Aspirin is filterable at the glomerulus, and so its concentration in Bowman's space is identical to that in peritubular plasma; moreover, because the pH of the glomerular filtrate is identical to that of peritubular plasma, the relative proportions of ASA$^-$ and ASA-H are also the same in the two fluids. As the filtered fluid flows along the tubule, water is reabsorbed, and this removal of solvent concentrates both ASA$^-$ and ASA-H, thereby creating lumen-to-plasma diffusion gradients favoring net reabsorption (exactly as described for urea). Since only ASA-H can penetrate the membrane to any great extent, only this form is reabsorbed. Simultaneously (and this is really the crucial point) secretion of hydrogen ions into the lumen lowers the luminal pH and favors, by mass action, the generation of ASA-H, which can then diffuse along its concentration gradient from lumen to peritubular plasma (Fig. 13). In other words, water reabsorption is one factor which helps create the concentration gradient required for passive reabsorption, but luminal acidification, by generating the diffusible form of the substance from the nondiffusible form, is even more important in creating the gradient.

But the story is even more interesting, for as we shall see in Chap. 9, the tubular fluid can be made alkaline rather than more acid under certain circumstances. This would shift the intraluminal reaction toward generation of ASA⁻ at the expense of ASA-H, and the resulting decrease in luminal ASA-H would, of course, reduce the gradient for net reabsorption. Indeed, luminal ASA-H might actually fall below peritubular-capillary plasma ASA-H, thereby establishing a gradient for net passive *secretion* of ASA-H rather than reabsorption. Thus, the net passive reabsorption of weak organic acids is inversely related to urine pH, and net passive secretion may be seen when the urine is alkaline.

Readers should have little difficulty applying these same concepts to the passive renal tubular handling of weak bases:

$$B + H^+ \rightleftharpoons BH^+$$

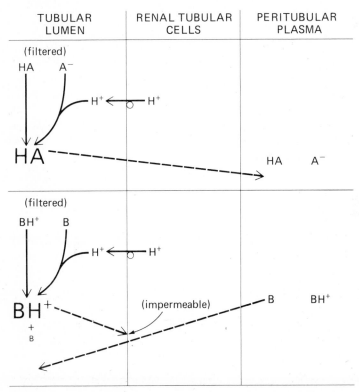

Figure 13 Acidification of the luminal fluid creates, by mass action, the gradients which drive net passive reabsorption (→) of weak acids (top) and net passive secretion (←) of weak bases (bottom).

When the tubular fluid is highly acidic, the generation of BH^+ from B is favored; the BH^+ cannot diffuse out of the lumen because of its charge, but the lowering of intraluminal B favors net passive secretion of B from peritubular-capillary plasma into the lumen. Conversely, when the urine is alkaline, generation of B within the lumen is favored, and a gradient is established for net passive reabsorption. Thus, weak bases are reabsorbed passively when the urine is alkaline but may be secreted (again, passively) when it is acid.

Finally, to make matters more complicated, it must now be emphasized that the description thus far has been in terms only of *passive* reabsorption and secretion of these substances. The fact is, as described earlier in this chapter, active secretory mechanisms exist in the proximal tubule for many weak acids and bases (specifically, for their anionic and cationic forms). Accordingly, they may be actively secreted into the proximal-tubular lumen followed by either passive reabsorption or passive secretion there and in the subsequent nephron segments, depending in part on urine flow rate but mainly upon the change in luminal pH occurring along the tubule.

Because so many medically used drugs are weak organic acids and bases, all these factors have important chemical implications. For example, if one wished to enhance the excretion of a drug which is a weak acid, one would attempt to alkalinize the urine; in contrast, acidification of the urine is desirable if one wished to prevent excretion of the drug. Of course, exactly the opposite would apply to weak organic bases. Increasing the urine flow would increase the excretion of both weak acids and bases. Finally, excretion could be reduced by interfering with any active proximal secretory pathway for the drug.

Study questions: **8** and **9**

Chapter 4

Renal Clearance

OBJECTIVES

The student understands the principles and applications of clearance technique.

1 Defines the term clearance
2 Knows which clearances are used to measure GFR and ERPF
3 Lists the data required for clearance calculation
4 Given data, calculates C_{in}, C_{PAH}, C_{urea}, $C_{glucose}$, C_{Na}
5 Given data, calculates reabsorptive T_m for glucose and secretory T_m for PAH
6 Given data, calculates rates of reabsorption of Na, protein, glucose, phosphate, and other substances not secreted
7 Knows how to estimate GFR from C_{urea} and describes the limitations
8 Describes the limitation of C_{Cr} as a measure of GFR
9 Predicts whether a substance has undergone net reabsorption or net secretion from its clearance relative to that of inulin
10 Constructs the curve relating steady-state P_{Cr} to C_{Cr} or P_{urea} to C_{urea}; predicts the changes in P_{Cr} and P_{urea} given a known change in GFR; knows the limitations of this analysis, particularly with regard to urea

When we described how inulin could be used to measure GFR, we were actually describing a technique known as clearance. We should like to explain this concept more fully and to reemphasize its usefulness in evaluating renal function.

DEFINITION

First, let us define the term. The _clearance_ of a substance is the _volume_ of _plasma_ from which that substance is _completely cleared_ by the kidneys _per unit time_. Every substance in the blood has its own distinct clearance value, and the units are always in volume of plasma per time. Inulin offers an excellent first example. Since all excreted inulin must come from the plasma, one can see that a certain volume of plasma loses its inulin while flowing through the kidney; i.e., a certain volume of plasma is "cleared" of inulin. For inulin, this volume is obviously equal to the GFR, since none of the inulin contained in the glomerular filtrate returns to the blood (inulin is not reabsorbed) and since none of the plasma that escapes filtration loses any of its inulin (inulin is not secreted). Therefore, a volume of plasma equal to the GFR has been completely cleared of inulin. This volume is termed the inulin clearance and is expressed as C_{In}. Accordingly,

$$C_{In} = GRF$$

What is the glucose clearance? Glucose is freely filtered at the glomerulus so that all the glucose contained in the glomerular filtrate is lost _initially_ from the plasma to the tubules. But, all of this filtered glucose is normally then reabsorbed; i.e., it is all returned to the plasma. The net result is that _no_ plasma ends up losing glucose; the clearance of glucose is _zero_.

What is the phosphate clearance in the example cited earlier? The filtered PO_4 equals 180 mmol/day. Is this the phosphate clearance? The answer is _no_. Clearance does _not_ designate a filtered mass. Indeed, it does not designate any mass; it is always a volume per time. The clearance of phosphate is defined as the volume of plasma completely cleared of phosphate per unit time. Is the clearance of phosphate, then, the GFR? Again the answer is _no_. Certainly, the filtered phosphate contained in the GFR is _temporarily_ lost from the plasma, but much of it is reabsorbed, in this example, 160 mmol/day, leaving only 20 mmol/day to be excreted in the urine. Is this the phosphate clearance?

Once again the answer is _no_. Clearance is not defined as mass excreted but rather as the volume of plasma supplying that mass per unit time. In other words, the phosphate clearance is the volume of plasma which supplies the excreted 20 mmol; it is this volume which is completely cleared of its phosphate. How much plasma has to be completely cleared of phosphate to supply the 20 mmol? We know from the data that the plasma phosphate concentration equals 1 mmol/L. Therefore, it would take

$$\frac{20 \text{ mmol/day}}{1 \text{ mmol/L}} = 20 \text{ L/day}$$

to supply the excreted phosphate. Clearance of a substance really answers the question: How much plasma must be completely cleared to supply the excreted mass of that substance? This is really synonymous with the formal definition of clearance given above.

BASIC FORMULA

It should be evident, therefore, that the basic clearance formula for any substance X is:

$$C_X = \frac{\text{mass of X excreted/time}}{P_X}$$
$$C_X = \frac{U_X V}{P_X}$$

where C_X = the clearance of substance X
 U_X = urine concentration of X
 V = urine volume per time
 P_X = arterial plasma concentration of X[1]

C_{In} is a measure of GFR simply because the volume of plasma completely cleared of inulin, i.e., the volume from which the excreted inulin comes, is equal to the volume of plasma filtered. C_{PO_4} must be less than C_{In} because much of the filtered phosphate is reabsorbed; therefore, less plasma was cleared of phosphate than of inulin.

Thus, the following generalization emerges: Whenever the clearance of a freely filterable substance is less than the inulin clearance, tubular reabsorption of that substance must have occurred. This is simply another way of stating that whenever the mass of a substance excreted in the urine is less than the mass filtered during the same period of time, tubular reabsorption must have occurred. The phrase "freely filterable" is essential in the above generalization. Protein serves as an excellent example. The

---

[1]In performing clearances, limb-vein blood may be used rather than arterial blood as long as the substances being studied are not synthesized or metabolized by the tissues of the limb.

clearance of protein in a normal person is essentially zero, obviously lower than the C_{In}. However, this does not prove that protein is reabsorbed; the major reason for the zero clearance is that the protein is not filtered. Accordingly, in order to compare inulin clearance to the clearance of any completely or partially protein-bound substance (calcium, for example), one must use the free plasma concentration of the substance, rather than the total plasma concentration, in the clearance formula.

Is the clearance of creatinine in humans higher or lower than that of inulin? The answer is higher. Like inulin, creatinine is freely filtered and not reabsorbed; therefore, a volume of plasma equal to that of the GFR (i.e., the C_{In}) is completely cleared of creatinine. But, in addition, a small amount of creatinine is secreted. Therefore, some plasma in addition to that filtered is cleared of its creatinine by means of tubular secretion. The clearance formula is precisely the same as that for any other substance.

$$C_{Cr} = \frac{U_{Cr}V}{P_{Cr}}$$

Another generalization emerges: Whenever the clearance of a substance is greater than the inulin clearance, tubular secretion of that substance must have occurred. Again, this is merely another way of stating that whenever the excreted mass exceeds the filtered mass, secretion must be occurring.

Another substance secreted by the proximal tubules is the organic anion para-aminohippurate (PAH). PAH is also filtered at the glomerulus, and, when its plasma concentration is fairly low, virtually all the PAH which escapes filtration is secreted. Since PAH is not reabsorbed, the net effect is that all the plasma supplying the nephrons is completely cleared of PAH. If PAH were completely cleared from all the plasma flowing through the *entire* kidney, then its clearance would measure the *total renal plasma flow* (TRPF). However, about 10 to 15 percent of the total renal plasma flow supplies nonsecreting portions of the kidneys, such as peripelvic fat, and this plasma cannot, therefore, lose its PAH by secretion. Accordingly, the PAH clearance actually measures the so-called *effective renal plasma flow* (ERPF) and is approximately 85 to 90 percent of the true *total* renal plasma flow. The clearance formula for PAH is, of course:

$$C_{PAH} = \frac{U_{PAH}V}{P_{PAH}}$$

Once we have measured the ERPF,[1] we can calculate easily the *effective renal blood flow* (ERBF):

$$\text{ERBF} = \frac{\text{ERPF}}{1 - V_c}$$

where V_c = the blood hematocrit, i.e., the fraction of blood occupied by erythrocytes.

It should be emphasized that C_{PAH} measures ERPF only when plasma PAH is fairly low. If plasma PAH were increased to a level so high that the PAH secretory T_m were exceeded, then PAH would not be completely removed from the plasma, and the use of its clearance as a measure of ERPF would be invalid. Another substance which is handled in a manner similar to PAH is Diodrast; accordingly, C_D is also a measure of ERPF.

Urea clearance C_{urea} can be determined by the usual formula:

$$C_{\text{urea}} = \frac{U_{\text{urea}}V}{P_{\text{urea}}}$$

Is the urea clearance higher or lower than inulin clearance? The answer is lower. Urea, like inulin, is freely filterable, but approximately 50 percent of filtered urea is reabsorbed; therefore, C_{urea} will be 50 percent of C_{In}. If the mass of urea reabsorbed were always exactly 50 percent of that filtered, could C_{urea} be used to estimate GFR? The answer is yes. One would merely multiply the C_{urea} by 2 to obtain a value equal to the GFR. Unfortunately, as described above, urea reabsorption varies between 40 and 60 percent of the filtered urea so that one cannot merely multiply by 2. Nonetheless, the clearance is easy to perform clinically and can be used as at least a crude indicator of glomerular function. The creatinine clearance is certainly a better way of evaluating GFR. But recall that, because of creatinine secretion, it is not completely accurate either.

To reiterate, whenever the clearance of a freely filterable substance is less than the simultaneously measured inulin clearance, reabsorption of that substance must have occurred; when its clearance is more than that

---

[1]To reiterate, C_{PAH} measures ERPF not TRPF because some PAH escapes filtration and secretion. However, we can measure the amount which has escaped simply by measuring the concentration of PAH in the renal venous plasma. We can then measure TRPF by using this value in the following equation:

$$\text{TRPF} = \frac{U_{\text{PAH}}V}{\text{arterial}_{\text{PAH}} - \text{renal venous}_{\text{PAH}}}$$

It should be evident that this equation is simply another example of the law of conservation of mass: What comes in at the renal artery must go out by the renal vein and urine combined.

of inulin, secretion must have occurred. Another way of stating these relationships without recourse to the term *clearance* was given earlier. The identity of these statements can be seen if one simply substitutes C_{In} for GFR in the equation

$$\text{Mass excreted} = \text{mass filtered} + (\text{mass secreted} - \text{mass reabsorbed})$$
$$(U_X V) \qquad\qquad (\text{GFR} \times P_X)$$
$$\text{or}$$
$$(C_{In} \times P_X)$$

Both are nothing more than the law of conservation of mass.

Note that reabsorption and secretion are not *directly measured* variables but are derived as a single value from the measurements of filtered and excreted masses. (Just move the term *mass filtered* to the left side of the equation to see this.) For this reason, if the mass excreted is greater than the mass filtered, this proves overall secretion by the tubules but does not disprove reabsorption; reabsorption might also have been present but masked by a greater rate of secretion. Similarly, proof of the presence of overall reabsorption, using clearance methods (excretion < filtration), does not disprove the possibility that secretion, too, is present but of lesser magnitude than reabsorption.

PLASMA CREATININE AND UREA CONCENTRATION AS INDICATORS OF GFR CHANGES

As described previously, the creatinine clearance is a close approximation of the GFR and is, therefore, a valuable clinical determination.

$$C_{Cr} = \frac{U_{Cr} V}{P_{Cr}}$$

In practice, however, it is far more common to measure plasma creatinine alone and to use this as an *indicator* of GFR. This approach is justified by the fact that most excreted creatinine gains entry to the tubule by filtration. If we ignore the small amount secreted, there should be an excellent inverse correlation between plasma creatinine and GFR, as shown by the following example: A normal person's plasma creatinine is 10 mg/L. It remains stable because each day the amount of creatinine produced is excreted. One day the GFR suddenly decreases permanently by 50 percent because of a blood clot in the renal artery. On that day the person filters only 50 percent as much creatinine as normal so that creatinine excretion is also reduced by 50 percent. (We are ignoring the small contribution of secreted creatinine.) Therefore, assuming no change in creatinine production, he or she goes into positive creatinine balance, and the plasma creatinine rises. But despite the persistent 50 percent GFR reduction, the plasma creatinine does not indefinitely continue to rise; rather, it stabilizes at 20 mg/L, i.e., after it has doubled. At this point he or she once again is able to excrete creatinine at the normal rate and so remains stable. The reason is that the 50 percent GFR reduction has been counterbalanced by the increase in plasma creatinine, and filtered creatinine is again normal.

Original normal state: Filtered creatinine = 10 mg/L × 180 L/day
= 1800 mg/day
New steady state: Filtered creatinine = 20 mg/L × 90 L/day
= 1800 mg/day

What if the GFR then fell to 30 L/day? Again creatinine retention would occur until a new steady state had been established, i.e., until he or she is again filtering 1800 mg/day. What would the new plasma creatinine be?

1800 mg/day = P_{Cr} × 30 L/day
P_{Cr} = 60 mg/L

It should now be clear why a single plasma creatinine is a reasonable indicator of GFR (Fig. 14). It is not completely accurate for three reasons: (1) Some creatinine is secreted. (2) There is no way of knowing exactly

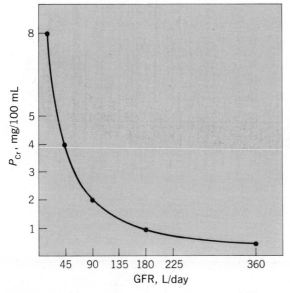

Figure 14 Steady-state relationship between GFR and plasma creatinine (assuming no creatinine is secreted).

what his or her original creatinine was when GFR was normal. (3) Creatinine production may not remain completely unchanged.

Since urea is also handled by filtration, the same type of analysis would indicate the measurement of plasma urea concentration and could serve as an indicator of GFR. However, it is much less accurate because the range of normal plasma urea concentration varies widely, depending upon protein intake and changes in tissue catabolism, and because urea is reabsorbed to a *variable* degree. The fact that it is reabsorbed would not interfere with its use as an indicator if the reabsorption were always a *fixed* percent of the filtered mass.

Study questions: **10** to **18**

Chapter 5

Renal Hemodynamics

OBJECTIVES

The student understands the control of renal hemodynamics.

1 States the formula relating flow, pressure, and resistance
2 Knows the normal rates of the GFR and RBF and defines filtration fraction
3 Defines autoregulation of RBF and GFR; states the condition in which "pure" autoregulation can be observed
4 Describes the role of the renal sympathetic nerves and states when their activity is increased
5 Describes how changes in filtration fraction occur
6 States the effect of angiotensin on renal arterioles
7 Describes two stimuli for increased renin secretion during hypotensive hemorrhage
8 States the adaptive value of the renal vasoconstriction induced by the renal nerves and angiotensin
9 States the effect of the renal nerves and angiotensin on renal prostaglandins and its significance
10 Defines distribution of flow (cortex-medulla and cortex-cortex)

The total blood flow to the kidneys in a typical adult is approximately 1.1 L/min. Thus, the kidneys receive 20 to 25 percent of the total cardiac output (5 L/min) even though their combined weight is less than 1 percent of the total body weight! Given a normal hematocrit of 0.45, the total renal plasma flow = 0.55×1.1 L/min = 605 mL/min. Recall that the GFR equals 125 mL/min. Therefore, of the 605 mL of plasma that enters the glomeruli via the afferent arterioles, $^{125}/_{605}$, or 20 percent, filters into Bowman's capsule, the remaining 480 mL passing via the efferent arterioles into the peritubular capillaries. This ratio is known as the *filtration fraction*.

Recall that the basic equation for blood flow through any organ is

$$\text{Organ blood flow} = \frac{\Delta P}{R}$$

where ΔP = mean arterial pressure minus venous pressure for that organ
R = resistance to flow through that organ

Recall also that, normally, the major determinant of resistance is the radii of the arterioles within that organ. It should be evident, therefore, that renal blood flow is determined mainly by the mean arterial pressure and the magnitude of renal arteriolar resistance.

MEAN ARTERIAL PRESSURE AND AUTOREGULATION

The renal circulation manifests quite markedly the phenomenon of autoregulation. The rate of blood flow through the kidney is relatively constant in the face of changes in mean arterial pressure—at least in the face of mean arterial pressures that range between 80 and 180 mmHg. Look again at the basic cardiovascular equation above. This equation predicts that if the pressure gradient is increased by 50 percent and resistance stays constant, blood flow will increase 50 percent. In the kidney, however, such is not the case. If one isolates a kidney experimentally and perfuses it with blood by means of a pump, one can demonstrate that a 50 percent increase in pressure gradient produces less than a 10 percent increase in blood flow. There is only one possible explanation: Resistance in the kidney does *not* stay constant as arterial pressure increases. Rather, resistance automatically increases. The renal arterioles constrict when the arterial pressure increases; therefore, blood flow remains relatively unchanged.

This entire discussion applies not only to RBF but to GFR, which also shows only small changes in the face of large changes in arterial pressure. There are several reasons for the fact that GFR, as well as RBF, is autoregulated. One of the most important is that the *afferent* arterioles are the major site of autoregulatory resistance changes in the face of arterial-pressure changes; accordingly, glomerular-capillary pressure (and, therefore, net filtration pressure) remains relatively unchanged.[1] For example, a rise in arterial pressure triggers enhanced afferent-arteriolar constriction, thereby increasing the pressure drop between the arteries and glomerular capillaries and preventing the transmission of the increased arterial pressure to the glomerulus.

What is the mechanism of autoregulation; i.e., how does an increase in renal arterial pressure elicit enhanced contraction of the smooth muscle of afferent arterioles, whereas a reduction in pressure elicits relaxation? One thing is for certain—the mechanism is completely intrarenal since it can be elicited in an isolated kidney perfused in vitro. That is about all that is certain, for the autoregulatory pathway has been the subject of intense controversy for many years. Renal physiologists have been loath to believe that the mechanism is probably the same as that found in other (nonrenal) autoregulating vascular beds, and they have attempted to explain it in terms of the unique architecture of the kidneys; for example, most recently as a chemical feedback from the macula densa to afferent arterioles at the juxtaglomerular apparatus. Unfortunately, neither this theory nor any other presently postulated seems able to explain autoregulation fully.

What is the adaptive value of autoregulation? As in any other organ, it helps ameliorate blood-flow changes in the face of arterial-pressure fluctuations, but it also serves a unique role in the kidney, namely the blunting of the large changes in solute and water excretion which could otherwise occur (because of large GFR changes) whenever arterial pressure changed. This is the adaptive value of GFR autoregulation. Recall that the normal net filtration pressure in the glomeruli is only about 5 to 6 mmHg. Accordingly, even relatively minor changes in arterial pressure could cause marked increases or decreases in glomerular-capillary pressure and GFR were not these changes effectively blunted by automatically elicited changes in afferent-arteriolar tonus.

Having pointed out the value of autoregulation, we must now emphasize three facts: (1) Autoregulation is not perfect. RBF and GFR *do change* when renal arterial pressure is changed, but they change to a much smaller degree than they would if autoregulation did not exist. (2) Autoregulation is virtually absent at mean arterial pressures below 70 mmHg and, therefore, cannot blunt GFR and RBF changes below this point. (3) Despite autoregulation, RBF and GFR *can be altered considerably,* even when the arterial pressure is within the autoregulatory range, by the factors to be described next—the sympathetic nervous system and the renin-angiotensin system.

[1]A second reason is described by Deen et al., 1974. (See Suggested Readings, Chap. 4.)

NEURAL CONTROL

In the above discussion of autoregulation, we set up artificial experimental conditions in which renal blood pressure could be changed without altering blood pressure in the other arteries of the body. In order to demonstrate autoregulation clearly, this is necessary because, when the systemic arterial pressure decreases in the *intact* organism, a second variable is brought into play. This variable is increased activity in the renal sympathetic nerves (and increased circulating epinephrine) reflexly mediated via the carotid sinus and aortic arch baroreceptors (Fig. 15). This sympathetic input causes renal arteriolar constriction (via α-adrenergic receptors), which decreases both RBF and GFR. Thus, although autoregulation blunts the *direct* effects on the kidney of changes in arterial pressure, *sympathetic reflexes* can cause changes in renal hemodynamics when systemic arterial pressure is altered.

What is the adaptive value of this reflex renal vasoconstriction? It is

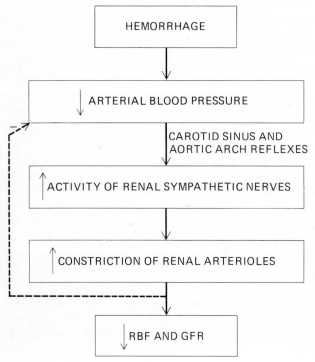

Figure 15 Pathway by which hypotension causes vasoconstriction mediated by the renal sympathetic nerves. Epinephrine, released from the adrenal medulla, also enhances renal vasoconstriction. The increased renal resistance helps to restore blood pressure (the negative-feedback loop) by contributing to increased total peripheral resistance.

simply one component of the overall control system for homeostatic regulation of arterial blood pressure. The renal vasoconstriction contributes to the rise in total peripheral resistance which helps restore the arterial blood pressure toward normal. But there is a second, less obvious way in which renal vasoconstriction helps raise blood pressure—the decrease in GFR and RBF result, as we shall see in a subsequent chapter, in a lowering of the excretion of sodium chloride and water; this has long-term consequences for regulation of blood volume and, thereby, arterial pressure.

In the description above, we saw that both GFR and RBF are decreased when sympathetic outflow to the kidneys increases. If sympa-

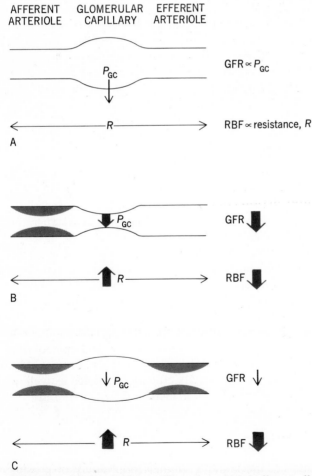

Figure 16 Effects of afferent (B) and combined afferent-efferent (C) arteriolar constriction on GFR and RBF. Adding efferent constriction lowers RBF still further (because total resistance is increased) but restores GFR toward normal. The ratio GFR/RBF is, therefore, increased.

thetic input were solely to the afferent arteriole, then the decreases in GFR and RBF induced by increased sympathetic tone would be approximately the same. However, both afferent and efferent arterioles are constricted when sympathetic tone is increased; therefore, GFR tends not to decrease as much as RBF. The reason for this is that, because the efferent arterioles lie beyond the glomerulus, an increase in their resistance tends to raise glomerular-capillary pressure—just the opposite of the effect of afferent-arteriolar constriction (see Fig. 16). In other words, increased sympathetic tone to the kidneys causes both GFR and RBF to decrease, but because GFR goes down less than RBF, the GFR/RBF ratio goes up. We shall make use of this fact in a subsequent chapter, when the control of salt and water excretion is described.

Finally, it should be emphasized that although this entire discussion has been in terms of the renal response to arterial hypotension, the same type of sympathetically mediated vasoconstriction can also be triggered by baroreceptors in the veins or cardiac chambers as well as by input from higher brain centers (for example, during heavy exercise or emotional situations).

ANGIOTENSIN

Norepinephrine and epinephrine are not the only vasoconstrictor agents to which the renal arterioles respond. Angiotensin is also a powerful vasoconstrictor, and the renal arterioles are quite sensitive to it. As described in Chap. 1, the plasma concentration of angiotensin is increased when the kidneys are stimulated to secrete more renin; accordingly, angiotensin-induced renal vasoconstriction can be expected whenever renin secretion is significantly elevated. The actual pathways mediating increased renin secretion will be described in detail in Chap. 7, but suffice it for present purposes to point out that two important stimuli are decreased arterial pressure and the renal sympathetic nerves. Thus, to return to our example of hemorrhage (Fig. 17), renal vasoconstriction in this situation is due not only to norepinephrine released from the renal nerves (and epinephrine from the adrenal medulla) but to angiotensin as well. This hormone, like norepinephrine and epinephrine, constricts efferent arterioles as well as afferent arterioles, and so it too produces an increased GFR/RBF ratio.

PROSTAGLANDINS

As pointed out in Chap. 1, the kidneys synthesize a variety of prostaglandins, including several which are potent vasodilators (and at least one which is a vasoconstrictor). Therefore, it has been tempting to speculate that the renal prostaglandins might serve as completely intrarenal local

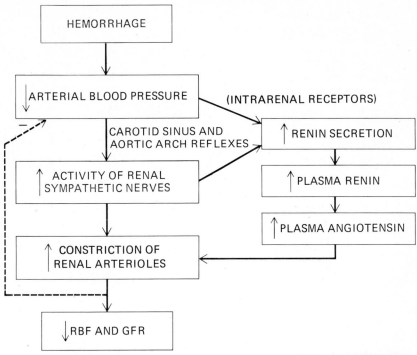

Figure 17 Contribution of angiotensin to renal vasoconstriction elicited by hemorrhage. This is simply Fig. 15 with the angiotensin pathway added. The mechanisms by which decreased arterial pressure (acting within the kidneys) and the sympathetic nerves stimulate renin release are described in Chap. 7.

modulators of renal blood flow in a variety of situations. The best documented role for the vasodilator prostaglandins in this regard is to "dampen" the vasoconstrictor effect of the renal nerves and angiotensin. The fact is that either an increased activity of the renal nerves or an increased plasma angiotensin stimulates the kidney to synthesize and release vasodilator prostaglandins; the end result is that much of the vasoconstrictor actions of norepinephrine and angiotensin are counteracted by the vasodilator action of the prostaglandins, and renal resistance changes much less than would otherwise have occurred (Fig. 18).

Thus, if we return once more to our example of hypotension due to hemorrhage, we see that three factors are reducing renal blood flow—the decreased blood pressure per se, the renal sympathetic nerves, and angiotensin; simultaneously, two factors are minimizing the fall—autoregulation and the prostaglandins, whose release is stimulated by the renal nerves and angiotensin. The net result is usually a modest increase in renal vascular resistance, leading to a modest decrease in RBF. The adaptive value of having such opposing inputs is to strike a balance be-

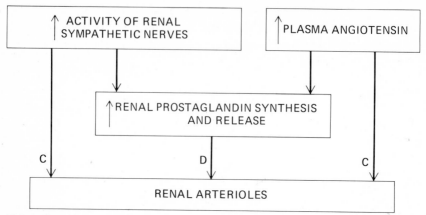

Figure 18 "Dampening" effect of prostaglandins on renal vasoconstriction induced by the renal nerves or angiotensin (C = constriction; D = dilation).

tween the requirement for an increased total peripheral resistance to maintain systemic arterial pressure (for the "benefit" of the heart and brain) and the likelihood of renal damage were renal vasoconstriction too severe. For example, an experimental animal given a drug which blocks prostaglandin synthesis and then subjected even to a modest hemorrhage may suffer rapidly occurring severe renal damage due to a profound reduction in renal blood flow.

OTHER POSSIBLE AGENTS

The renal vasculature is sensitive to many other normally occurring substances, including antidiuretic hormone, histamine, bradykinin, and adenosine. But whether any of these substances actually participates in the control of the renal circulation in health or disease is unclear.

INTRARENAL DISTRIBUTION OF BLOOD FLOW

Total renal blood flow can be measured readily either by clearance techniques or by more direct methods, such as flow probes. However, measurement of *regional* blood flows within the kidney has proven to be quite difficult. One well-established fact is that the cortex receives more than 90 percent of the total renal blood flow. The paucity of medullary blood flow (its adaptive value for urine concentration will be discussed later) is due to the resistance offered by the vasa recta, but it is not yet possible to quantitate the contributions of the multiple factors (vessel length, blood viscosity, neural tone, chemical mediators, etc.) which cause the resistance in the vasa recta to be higher than in the other intrarenal vessels.

Even more difficult to analyze is the relative distribution of blood flow within the cortex between the juxtamedullary and outer cortical nephrons. It does seem clear that differences exist and are subject to physiological control. (The possible significance of this phenomenon for the renal handling of sodium and water is discussed in Chap. 7.) The controlling factors have not been clearly determined, but differences in sympathetic outflow to the arterioles of the outer and juxtamedullary areas of the cortex, as well as differences in autoregulatory responses and prostaglandin-synthesis capabilities of these areas all may be involved.

Study questions: **19** and **20**

Chapter 6

Basic Renal Processes for Sodium, Chloride, and Water

OBJECTIVES

The student understands the basic renal processes for sodium, chloride, and water.

1 Calculates or lists the quantities of sodium, chloride, and water normally filtered, reabsorbed, and excreted per day

2 Describes the nature (active or passive) of the process for each substance and the interrelationships between them, i.e., the forces involved; defines transtubular PD and gives its orientation in the different nephron segments

3 Describes the pathway followed by the transported fluid; defines tight junctions and intercellular spaces; states how increased interstitial hydraulic pressure can lead to "back-leakage" in the proximal tubule

4 Describes the mechanism of action of osmotic diuretics; distinguishes osmotic diuresis from water diuresis

5 States the fluid osmolarity and relative water permeability in each nephron segment during water diuresis and antidiuresis

6 Lists the percentages of sodium and water reabsorbed by each nephron segment during antidiuresis and water diuresis

7 Describes the countercurrent multiplier system for urine concentration; states the transport and permeability characteristics of the ascending and descending limbs, the distal tubules and the collecting ducts

8 States the net loss or gain of solute and water for the two limbs of the loop and the collecting duct; states the action of ADH and the nephron sites on which it acts

9 Describes the medullary circulation and its functioning as a countercurrent exchanger

10 States how changes in medullary blood flow or loop flow rates may impede concentration of the urine

11 Describes the obligatory relationships between sodium and water excretion; states how the nephron segments differ in their ability to develop transtubular sodium gradients

Table 1 was a typical balance sheet for water; Table 6 is the same for sodium. The excretion of sodium via the skin and gastrointestinal tract is normally quite small but may increase markedly during severe sweating, burns, vomiting, diarrhea, or hemorrhage.

Control of the renal excretion of sodium and water constitutes the most important mechanism for the regulation of body sodium and water. The excretory rates of these substances can be varied over an extremely wide range. For example, a consumer of gross amounts of salt may ingest 20 to 25 g of sodium chloride per day, whereas a patient on a low-salt diet may ingest only 50 mg. The normal kidney can readily alter its excretion of salt over this range. Similarly, urinary water excretion can be varied physiologically from approximately 400 mL/day to 25 L/day depending upon whether one is lost in the desert or participating in a beer-drinking contest.

Sodium, chloride, and water are all freely filterable at the glomerulus and undergo considerable tubular reabsorption—normally, more than 99 percent (see Table 4)—but no tubular secretion. Most renal energy utili-

Table 6   Normal Routes of Sodium Chloride Intake and Loss

Route	g/day
Intake	
Food	10.5
Output	
Sweat	0.25
Feces	0.25
Urine	10.0
Total output	10.5

zation goes to accomplish this enormous reabsorptive task. The major tubular mechanisms for reabsorption of these substances can be summarized by three generalizations which apply to all nephron segments with the exception of the loop of Henle: (1) The reabsorption of sodium is an active process; i.e., it is carrier-mediated, requires an energy supply, and can occur against an electrochemical gradient. (2) The reabsorption of chloride is primarily by diffusion and depends upon the active reabsorption of sodium. (3) The reabsorption of water also is passive and depends mainly upon the active reabsorption of sodium. Thus, active tubular sodium reabsorption is the primary force which results in reabsorption of chloride and water as well.

As mentioned above, the loop of Henle constitutes an exception to the generalizations. Present evidence suggests that the descending limb does not reabsorb sodium or chloride at all, and in the ascending limb, the first two generalizations given above are reversed; i.e., chloride reabsorption is the primary, active process, and sodium reabsorption is by diffusion, dependent upon the active chloride movement. The third generalization still holds in that water reabsorption by the loop of Henle is passive and dependent upon active ion transport except that, in this case, the actively transported ion is chloride rather than sodium.

In describing next the mechanisms by which ion-ion and ion-water movements are coupled, we shall do so in terms of active sodium transport, since this process is the key event in most nephron segments. Finally, it should at least be noted at this point that reabsorption of sodium, chloride, and water is intimately associated with reabsorption of the other major anion of plasma—bicarbonate—but this additional complexity will not be described until Chap. 9.

SODIUM-WATER COUPLING

We previously described in Chap. 2 the basic pathway for sodium reabsorption; let us do so again, this time emphasizing how the passive reabsorption of water is coupled to it. The key fact to keep in mind is that sodium reabsorption creates the osmotic gradient between lumen and interstitial fluid required to produce net diffusion of water in the same direction.

Figure 19 summarizes events in the proximal tubule, other nephron segments being at least qualitatively similar. Since the concentrations of all crystalloids are essentially identical in plasma and in Bowman's capsular fluid, no significant transtubular concentration differences exist at the beginning of the proximal tubule for sodium, chloride, or water. As the fluid flows down the tubule, sodium is actively reabsorbed. Recall that luminal sodium ions enter the cell by facilitated diffusion along the electrochemical gradient created by the Na-K-ATPase–dependent active

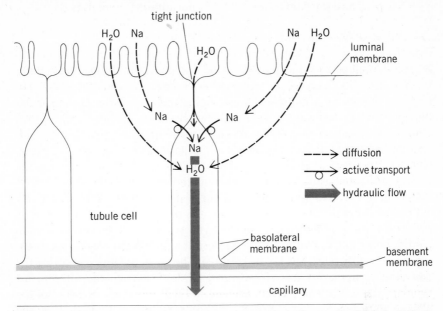

Figure 19 Pathway for sodium and water reabsorption in the proximal tubule. The active Na step occurs all along the basolateral membrane, not just at the segment below the tight junction.

transport of sodium across the basolateral membrane into the intercellular spaces. The removal of sodium from the lumen lowers total luminal osmolarity (i.e., raises water concentration) and simultaneously raises the osmolarity (lowers the water concentration) in the intercellular spaces. This osmotic gradient from lumen to intercellular space causes net diffusion of water from the lumen across the cell membranes and/or tight junctions into the intercellular spaces.

Just how much net osmosis will occur under any given lumen-to-interstitium osmotic gradient is determined by the permeability to water of the cell membranes and tight junctions. The proximal tubule, for example, is so permeable to water that very small gradients suffice to move large quantities of water. In contrast, the distal convoluted tubule is so impermeable to water that almost no water reabsorption occurs no matter how large the osmotic gradient. Finally, and perhaps most important, the water permeability of nephron segments beyond the distal convoluted tubule is not fixed but is subject to physiological control.

Thus far we have been describing the movements of sodium and water out of the lumen and into the interstitial fluid of the intercellular spaces. What causes this reabsorbed fluid to move from interstitial fluid into peritubular capillaries? It is, simply, the net balance of hydraulic and oncotic pressures acting across the capillaries.

Net pressure for fluid movement into peritubular capillaries is

$$P_{net} = P_{Int} + \pi_{PC} - P_{PC} - \pi_{Int}$$

where the subscripts Int and PC stand for interstitium and peritubular capillary, respectively. This is the second time we have dealt with capillary dynamics in the kidney, the first being the discussion of glomerular filtration. It must be emphasized that the concepts are identical, but, of course, the locations are different. Glomerular dynamics involve the balance of forces between the glomerular capillaries and Bowman's capsule, whereas the peritubular forces are between the interstitium and the peritubular capillaries (Table 7). Whereas the net driving pressure across the glomeruli always favors filtration out of the capillaries into Bowman's capsule, the net driving pressure across the peritubular capillaries always favors net movement into the capillaries (reabsorption). The major reason for the latter fact is twofold: (1) The peritubular-capillary hydraulic pressure is generally quite low (10 to 15 mmHg) because the blood entering the peritubular capillaries has already had to flow through the afferent arterioles, glomeruli, and efferent arterioles. (2) The oncotic pressure of the plasma entering the peritubular capillaries is higher than that of the plasma entering the glomeruli because the plasma proteins are concentrated by loss of protein-free filtrate during passage through the glomerular capillaries. (Early peritubular-capillary oncotic pressure is, therefore, identical to end-glomerular-capillary oncotic pressure.)

To reiterate, the final step in fluid reabsorption is bulk flow from interstitium (intercellular spaces) into peritubular capillaries. One of the factors favoring this movement is, as we have seen (Table 7), the hydraulic pressure in the intercellular spaces. A crucial new fact is that this hy-

Table 7   Estimated Forces Involved in Peritubular-Capillary Reabsorption
(i.e., Movement of Fluid from Interstitium into Capillaries)*

Forces	mmHg
1 Favoring reabsorption	
a Interstitial hydraulic pressure, P_{Int}	7
b Oncotic pressure in peritubular capillaries, π_{PC}	35
2 Opposing reabsorption	
a Hydraulic pressure in peritubular capillaries, P_{PC}	11
b Interstitial oncotic pressure, π_{Int}	6
3 Net pressure for reabsorption (1 − 2)	25

*The values for peritubular-capillary hydraulic and oncotic pressures are for the early portions of the capillary. The oncotic pressure, of course, decreases as protein-free fluid enters it, i.e., as absorption occurs, but would not go below 25 mmHg (the value of arterial plasma) even if all fluid originally filtered at the glomerulus were absorbed.

draulic pressure may, at the same time, produce some "backward" movement of reabsorbed fluid, i.e., bulk flow of intercellular fluid through the tight junctions between cells and back into the lumen. Such back-leakage, of course, reduces the *net* reabsorption of sodium and water, a point to which we shall return in the next chapter.

SODIUM-CHLORIDE COUPLING

How is the passive reabsorption of chloride coupled to the active transport of sodium? There are at least two mechanisms responsible for this coupling. The first mechanism is precisely the same as that previously described for urea. As water moves out of the tubule (secondary to sodium transport), all solutes in the tubule not subject to active transport will increase in concentration. By this means, a chloride transtubular *concentration gradient* is established, which acts as a driving force for chloride reabsorption by passive diffusion. (You should now recognize that the reabsorption of urea, just as that of chloride, is indirectly coupled to sodium transport via the latter's effect on water reabsorption.)

The second mechanism coupling passive chloride reabsorption to active sodium transport is the *electric potential difference* (PD) which exists across the tubular epithelium. In all nephron segments, with the exception of the loop of Henle (and probably also the later portions of the proximal tubule), the tubular lumen is negatively charged compared to the interstitial fluid. The magnitude of this lumen-negative PD varies throughout the tubule, ranging from 0 to -4 mV in the early proximal tubule to -40 to -60 mV in the distal tubule. One major contributing factor to this potential is undoubtedly the active reabsorption of sodium. Just on an intuitive level, it should be evident that the active transport of positively charged sodium ions across the epithelium tends to leave the inside of the lumen negatively charged.[1] A systematic analysis of the precise origins of this transtubular PD is beyond the scope of this presentation. What is more important for present purposes is the fact that this PD exists, is contributed to by active sodium transport, and constitutes a driving force for passive chloride reabsorption.

We have, then, both an electric and a chemical (i.e., concentration) difference favoring passive chloride reabsorption. In the proximal tubule, where the PD is very small (and may actually be slightly lumen-positive in its late portions), the concentration difference created by sodium-coupled water transport is most important. In the distal tubules and collecting ducts a very large PD exists and constitutes the major driving force for

---

[1]This statement assumes that sodium "pumps" in the renal tubule are rheogenic; i.e., they directly separate charge. Such is the case, for they are definitely not classical 1:1 Na^+-K^+ exchangers. This question will be dealt with in Chap. 8.

chloride movement. In both cases, however, the chloride movement is passive and is ultimately dependent upon active sodium reabsorption.

It should be possible for the reader to guess what the situation is in the ascending loop of Henle. In the ascending loop, chloride transport is the active primary event and causes the lumen to be positively charged relative to the peritubular fluid, and this constitutes a driving force for the passive reabsorption of sodium.

With these generalizations as guides, let us now discuss some of the distinct characteristics of the individual nephron segments relative to salt and water handling.

PROXIMAL TUBULE

The proximal tubule is the site of greatest sodium and water reabsorption. Approximately 65 percent of the total filtered sodium and water is reabsorbed by the time the fluid has reached the end of the proximal tubule. Its water permeability is always very great, so passive water reabsorption keeps pace with active sodium reabsorption.[1] What, therefore, is the concentration of sodium at the end of the proximal tubule? The answer is: almost equal to the plasma sodium concentration. It is true that 65 percent of the mass of sodium filtered has been reabsorbed but so has almost 65 percent of the filtered water. Therefore, the concentration of sodium, as opposed to the mass, remains virtually unchanged during fluid passage through the proximal tubule.

The above paragraph (and, indeed, the entire preceding discussion) implies that sodium is the only factor determining the osmotic gradient for net water reabsorption from the proximal tubule. This is, of course, an oversimplification, since any actively reabsorbed substance can, theoretically, contribute to a lowering of luminal osmolarity and, thereby, to a facilitation of water reabsorption; sodium is preeminent because it is by far the most plentiful solute and because its reabsorption drives the second most plentiful, chloride. The only other substance present in the glomerular filtrate in high concentration is bicarbonate; as we shall see in Chap. 9, bicarbonate reabsorption in the proximal tubule is an active process and more than keeps pace with sodium and water reabsorption; i.e., more than 65 percent is reabsorbed by the proximal tubule. Because of this, its concentration in the lumen falls below that in the plasma, and this

---

[1]Just how high the permeability of the proximal tubular epithelium is to water remains the subject of controversy because the overall lumen-interstitium osmotic gradient isn't known (the osmolarity in the lumen is known, but that in the intercellular spaces is not). The most recent estimate is that only 1 mosmol/L difference between lumen and intercellular space can account for most water reabsorption by the proximal tubule.

contributes to water reabsorption.[1] The proximally reabsorbed organic solutes described earlier in Chap. 3 (glucose, amino acids, citrate, lactate, etc.) also contribute, since their luminal concentrations may fall well below those in the plasma (often all the way to zero); however, recall that they are mainly co-transported with sodium so that their effect on water reabsorption ultimately is ascribable to sodium reabsorption.[2]

What is the osmolarity of the fluid at the end of the proximal tubule compared to plasma? This is, of course, merely the sum of all the different solute concentrations. Sodium is essentially the same as in plasma, as stressed in preceding paragraphs; chloride is slightly higher (since, given the forces driving its reabsorption, it must lag a little behind water); bicarbonate is somewhat lower, as described in the previous paragraph; some solutes (like glucose) are lower, whereas others (like urea) are higher. The end result is that the total osmolarity at the end of the proximal tubule is always essentially the same as that of the plasma. This, of course, is not just fortuitous but must be the case, given the extremely high permeability of the proximal tubule to water; i.e., water reabsorption always occurs at a rate which keeps the luminal osmolarity only very slightly less than that of the plasma.

To summarize, during passage through the proximal tubule, approximately 65 percent of the sodium, chloride, and water are reabsorbed, but the sodium concentration and osmolarity of the fluid remain essentially the same as in plasma. This fact raises an interesting question: If sodium concentration is approximately plasmalike throughout the proximal tubule, how do we know that sodium reabsorption is an active process? To prove active transport, we must demonstrate net transport against an electrochemical gradient; yet the proximal tubule has only a small transtubular electric gradient, and we normally find no concentration gradient. Assuming that sodium transport really is active, then the reason that no concentration gradient is normally created is that water reabsorption keeps up with sodium. We must create an experimental situation in which water movement is retarded; in such a case, sodium reabsorption will get well ahead of water reabsorption, intraluminal sodium concentration will fall, and active sodium transport will have been demonstrated. This condition occurs in the presence of an osmotic diuretic.

---

[1]As pointed out in Chap. 1, the proximal tubule is not homogenous along its entire length, and its different portions manifest quite different relative reabsorptive rates for chloride and bicarbonate. This may influence proximal fluid reabsorption in complex ways, which are not dealt with in this book but which in no way alter our working generalization concerning the primary importance of active sodium reabsorption.

[2]In our description in this chapter of sodium reabsorption by the proximal tubule, we ignored the role of the solutes, since only a small fraction of sodium movement is in association with them.

An *osmotic diuretic* is a substance which retards water (and sodium) reabsorption merely because of its osmotic contribution to the tubular fluid. Recall that sodium, chloride, and bicarbonate normally constitute most of the osmotically active solute in plasma. Let us alter the situation by administering to a dog large amounts of the sugar mannitol so that its plasma concentration equals 100 mosmol/L. Mannitol is freely filtered at the glomerulus but is not reabsorbed. In the first portion of the proximal tubule, therefore, mannitol will contibute 100 mosmol/L. As sodium is actively reabsorbed, the total osmolarity of the proximal-tubular fluid begins to decrease, and water, therefore, passively follows the sodium. However, because the mannitol cannot be reabsorbed, its concentration increases as water is reabsorbed. This type of concentrating effect has been previously described for chloride and for urea and obviously will apply to any solute whose reabsorption is slower than that of water. The crucial difference between our experimental conditions and the normal state is that the normally present "lagging" solutes either are present in low concentrations or, like chloride, follow closely behind the water. The mannitol, in contrast, is present in a very large concentration and is not reabsorbed at all. Accordingly, as its concentration rises as a result of water reabsorption, its osmotic presence retards the further reabsorption of water. Thus, passive water movement is prevented from keeping up with active sodium transport. The result is that sodium concentration in the lumen decreases significantly below plasma sodium concentration, and proof of net transport against a concentration gradient is obtained.

We would not have burdened the reader with this analysis if our sole purpose were to show how the active nature of proximal sodium transport was proven. Far more important for clinical medicine is the fact that osmotic diuresis occurs in several disease states, including diabetes mellitus. Glucose is normally completely reabsorbed in the proximal tubule. But in the patient with uncontrolled diabetes mellitus, the filtered load may exceed the glucose T_m, and large quantities of glucose may remain unreabsorbed in the proximal tubule. Just like mannitol in the above example, the presence of this glucose retards water reabsorption and causes an osmotic diuresis. In such a patient, the filtered load of the ketone bodies, acetoacetate and β-hydroxybutyrate, may also exceed the T_m's for these substances so that they also contribute to the osmotic diuresis.

In our discussion of osmotic diuresis we have emphasized the poor reabsorption and increased excretion of water which occurs. Less easy to understand is the fact that osmotic diuretics cause the excretion of large quantitites of sodium (and chloride) as well as of water. The major reason for this phenomenon illustrates another important characteristic of renal sodium transport: Simultaneously with the *active* transport of sodium out of the tubule, there are occurring quite large fluxes of sodium in both directions by simple diffusion, since the tubule is quite permeable to sodium. But is there a *net diffusional flux* into or out of the proximal tubule? Normally there is very little, since there is no significant transtubular concentration difference for sodium and since the electric potential difference across the proximal tubule is quite small. Therefore, the opposing diffusional fluxes of sodium simply cancel each other out, leaving only the outwardly directed *active* sodium-transport pathway to account for overall *net* sodium movement. However, in the presence of an osmotic diuretic, this situation is altered; because the osmotic diuretic retards water reabsorption, active sodium reabsorption causes the intratubular sodium concentration to decrease as described above. As a result there is a sodium concentration gradient favoring *net* diffusion of sodium from interstitial fluid to lumen. (We are speaking here of sodium *diffusion,* not of the back-leakage by *bulk flow* mentioned earlier.) This net passive influx opposes the active outflux, and so the *overall net* removal of sodium from the proximal-tubular lumen is diminished. This is one of the reasons that osmotic diuretics such as mannitol (or glucose in the diabetic) induce the excretion of large quantities of sodium (and chloride) as well as water. The impression should not be given that osmotic diuretics inhibit water and electrolyte reabsorption in the proximal tubule only. In fact, major inhibition occurs in the loop of Henle also (although the mechanism is not exactly the same).

LOOP OF HENLE

The loops of Henle normally reabsorb approximately 25 percent of the filtered sodium and chloride and 15 percent of the filtered water. What percentages of the filtered sodium and water, therefore, enter the distal tubule? The answer is: 10 and 20 percent, respectively, since one must add the quantities reabsorbed by the loop to those already reabsorbed by the proximal tubule to obtain the total quantities unreabsorbed prior to the distal tubule.

As mentioned earlier, the reabsorption of sodium, chloride, and water in the ascending loop is unusual in that chloride is the active process, which secondarily induces passive reabsorption of sodium. This explains why certain of the drugs used clinically to block sodium chloride reabsorption act mainly on the loop, whereas others do not. The specific interactions between sodium, chloride, and water are complex, and we shall return to them in a subsequent section, since they are so tied up with events in more distal segments. For the moment, it is sufficient to emphasize that the loop, unlike the proximal tubule, *reabsorbs considerably more solute than water.*

It is very likely that the macula densa, the junction between ascending loop and distal convoluted tubule, has functional characteristics similar to those of the ascending loop.

DISTAL TUBULE AND COLLECTING DUCT

Sodium and chloride reabsorption continues along the distal tubules and collecting ducts so that the final urine normally contains less than 1 percent of the total filtered sodium and chloride. (More important than this vague single value—"less than 1 percent"—is the fact that the exact number changes, depending upon the individual's salt balance, as we shall see in the next chapter.)

What about reabsorption of water? The water permeability of the early distal tubule (that portion corresponding to the distal convoluted tubule) is extremely low and unchanging.[1] Accordingly, almost no water is reabsorbed during passage of fluid through it. In contrast, the water permeability of the late distal tubules and the collecting ducts is subject to physiological control (see below) and may vary from extremely low to fairly high (although never as high as that of the proximal tubule).

Let us now combine this information on salt reabsorption and water permeability in following the changes in luminal sodium concentration and osmolarity along the distal tubule and collecting ducts. First, recall that, because more solute than water was reabsorbed in the loop, both the sodium concentration and osmolarity of the fluid entering the distal tubule are well below those of plasma. (The discrepancy is less for osmolarity than for sodium because, as described in Chap. 3, another major solute—urea—is added in the loop.) As fluid flows through the early distal tubule, sodium chloride reabsorption proceeds, but virtually no water is reabsorbed, despite the large osmotic gradient, because of the epithelium's low water permeability. The result is some further lowering of the osmolarity.

Beyond the early distal tubule, i.e., in the late distal tubule and the collecting duct system, the way in which osmolarity changes as the fluid flows along the tubule depends mainly upon the water permeability of the tubule. If the water permeability is very great, so much water is reabsorbed from the late distal tubules and cortical collecting tubules that the luminal fluid once more equilibrates with the plasma in the peritubular capillaries surrounding these structures, i.e., becomes isoosmotic (300 mosmol/L). After equilibrium has occurred, these segments behave

---

[1]Until recently it was not recognized that many micropuncture samples thought to be collected from the distal convoluted tubule were, in fact, from the initial collecting tubule, the so-called late distal tubule (see Table 2). This led to erroneous views concerning the water permeability of the distal convoluted tubule.

analogously to the proximal tubule, reabsorbing approximately equivalent amounts of solute and water. In contrast, when water permeability is low, the hypoosmotic fluid entering the late distal tubule may become even more hypoosmotic as it flows along the tubule, and sodium reabsorption continues, unaccompanied by equivalent water reabsorption.

The water permeability of the rest of the medullary collecting ducts shows the same variability as that of the cortical collecting tubules. Thus, in the presence of low permeability, the highly dilute fluid delivered from the cortical collecting tubules remains dilute as it flows through the medullary collecting ducts. In contrast, when the water permeability of the collecting ducts is very great, the isoosmotic fluid leaving the cortical collecting tubules is progressively concentrated in its passage through the medullary collecting ducts. This should come as a surprise since, on the basis of what has been so far described, one ought to conclude that the fluid would merely remain isoosmotic. The explanation will be given in the next section.

The major determinant of water permeability in the late distal tubules and the entire cortical and medullary collecting-duct system is the hormone known as vasopressin, or antidiuretic hormone (ADH). The second name describes the effect of the hormone's action—antidiuresis (i.e., against a high urine volume).[1] In the absence of ADH the tubular water permeability is very low, but sodium reabsorption may proceed normally because ADH (at least in physiological concentrations) has no significant effect on sodium reabsorption; thus, water is unable to follow and remains in the tubule to be excreted as a large volume of urine. On the other hand, in the presence of maximum amounts of ADH, the tubular water permeability is very great, and the final urine volume is small—less than 1 percent of the total filtered water. Of course, the tubular response to ADH is not all-or-none, like an action potential, but shows graded increases as the plasma concentration of ADH is increased over a certain range, thus permitting fine adjustments of water permeability and excretion.[2]

ADH exerts its action by stimulating the intracellular generation of cyclic AMP (via the adenylate cyclase system). Just how the increased cyclic AMP then increases water permeability is still not clear, but it most likely involves an increase in the number of membrane "pores" through which water can diffuse. Since such "pores" reflect the arrangement of

[1]The first name, vasopressin, denotes the fact that, when present in very high concentrations (attainable in certain disease states), this hormone constricts arterioles and, thereby, increases the arterial blood pressure.

[2]It is quite likely that ADH also induces increased intrarenal synthesis and release of prostaglandins, perhaps from the interstitial cells of the medulla. Prostaglandin then partially opposes the permeability-enhancing effect of ADH. Thus, via this sequence, ADH indirectly exerts a negative-feedback influence over its own effect. Abnormal prostaglandin synthesis (in either direction) may well account for the altered tubular responsiveness to ADH seen in certain renal diseases.

the membranes' integral proteins, it is likely that these proteins are the ultimate target molecules for the system.

It should now be easy to understand how the kidneys produce a final urine having the same osmolarity as that of plasma or one having a lower osmolarity than plasma (hypoosmotic urine), the latter occurring whenever water reabsorption lags behind solute reabsorption, i.e., when plasma ADH is reduced (this is known as *water diuresis*). In this regard, it is worth reemphasizing that, even when virtually no water reabsorption occurs beyond the loop of Henle because of an absence of ADH, the reabsorption of sodium is not retarded to any great extent; therefore, intraluminal sodium concentration can be lowered almost to zero in these nephron segments. Recall that the proximal tubule behaves very differently from this when its water reabsorption is blocked, in this case by the presence of an osmotic diuretic; under such conditions net sodium reabsorption is also greatly reduced because of the passive back-leak of sodium from interstitium to lumen. This does not occur to any great extent in the distal tubule and collecting duct because these segments are so much less permeable to sodium; i.e., passive (diffusional) fluxes are very low compared to the rate of active reabsorption. Accordingly, in comparison with the proximal tubule, extremely large transtubular gradients for sodium can be achieved by active reabsorption in these segments.

How can the kidneys ever produce a hyperosmotic urine, i.e., a urine having an osmolarity greater than that of plasma? For this to occur does not water reabsorption have to "get ahead" of solute reabsorption? How can this happen if water reabsorption is always secondary to solute, particularly salt, reabsorption? It would seem that if our generalizations are not to be violated, then the kidneys cannot produce a hyperosmotic urine. Yet, as we have mentioned, they do. Indeed, the final urine may be as concentrated as 1400 mosmol/L compared with a plasma osmolarity of 300 mosmol/L. Moreover, this concentrated urine is produced without violating the generalization that water reabsorption is always passive.

URINE CONCENTRATION: THE MEDULLARY COUNTERCURRENT SYSTEM

The ability of the kidneys to produce concentrated urine is not merely an academic problem. It is a major determinant of one's ability to survive without water. The human kidney can produce a maximal urinary concentration of 1400 mosmol/L. The urea, sulfate, phosphate, and other waste products (plus the small number of nonwaste ions) which must be excreted each day amount to approximately 600 mosmol. Therefore, the water required for their excretion constitutes an obligatory water loss and equals:

$$\frac{600 \text{ mosmol/day}}{1400 \text{ mosmol/L}} = 0.429 \text{ L/day} = \textit{obligatory urine loss/d}.$$

As long as the kidneys are functioning, excretion of this volume of urine will occur, despite the absence of water intake. In a sense, a person lacking access to water may literally urinate to death due to fluid depletion. If we could produce a urine with an osmolarity of 6000 mosmol/L, then only 100 mL of water need be lost obligatorily each day, and survival time would be greatly expanded. A desert rodent, the kangaroo rat, does just that. This animal never even drinks water because the water produced by oxidation is ample for its needs.

Countercurrent Multiplication

The kidneys produce concentrated urine by a complex interaction of events involving the collecting ducts and the so-called countercurrent multiplier system residing in the loop of Henle. Let us look first at events in the loop and then integrate them with those in the collecting ducts. Recall that the loop of Henle, which is interposed between the proximal and distal tubules, is a hairpin loop extending into the renal medulla. Let us list the critical characteristics of this loop:

   1   As described in Chap. 1, the ascending limb of the loop (i.e., the limb leading to the distal tubule) is not a structurally homogenous segment. It is very thin from the bend in the loop up to the outer medulla (only long loops have this thin ascending portion) where it becomes much thicker. This structural difference reflects functional differences as well. However, for simplicity, we initially present the physiological characteristics of the thicker portion as though they apply to the entire ascending limb. The ascending limb *actively* transports chloride out of the tubular lumen into the surrounding interstitium; i.e., it reabsorbs it. It is also fairly permeable to sodium (and chloride). Therefore, the active chloride transport causes the passive movement of sodium out of the lumen, and we shall refer to the overall process as sodium chloride transport. However, the ascending limb is always quite impermeable to water so that water cannot follow the sodium chloride.
   2   The descending limb of the loop (i.e., the limb into which drains fluid from the proximal tubule) does *not actively* transport either chloride or sodium. It is the only tubular segment that does not. Moreover, it has a very great permeability to water but is relatively impermeable to the ions.

Keeping these characteristics in mind, imagine the loop of Henle filled with a stationary column of fluid supplied by the proximal tubule. At first, the concentration everywhere would be 300 mosmol/L, since fluid leaving the proximal tubule is isoosmotic to plasma.

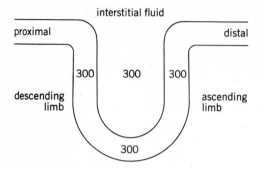

Now let the active pump in the ascending limb transport sodium chloride into the interstitium until a limiting gradient (say 200 mosmol/L) is established between ascending-limb fluid and interstitium.

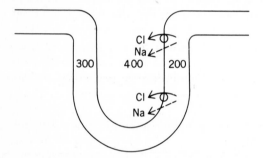

A limiting gradient is reached because the ascending limb is relatively permeable to chloride. Accordingly, passive back flux into the lumen counterbalances active outflux, and a steady-state limiting gradient is established.

Given the great permeability of the descending limb to water, there is a net diffusion of water[1] out of the descending limb and into the in-

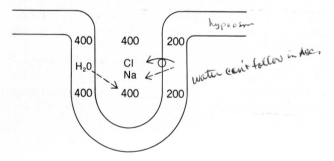

[1]The descending limb is not completely impermeable to sodium and chloride. Accordingly, some of these ions diffuse into the loop simultaneously with water movement out of the loop. For simplicity, we ignore this additional complexity. (See Kokko, 1974, in Suggested Readings for Chap. 6.)

terstitium until the osmolarities are equal. The interstitial osmolarity is maintained at 400 mosmol/L during this equilibration because of continued sodium chloride transport out of the ascending limb.

Note that the osmolarities of the descending limb and interstitium are equal and both are higher than that of the ascending limb. So far we have held the fluid stationary in the loop, but, of course, it is actually continuously flowing. Let us look at what occurs under conditions of flow. We shall simplify the analysis by assuming that flow through the loop, on the one hand, and ion and water movements, on the other, occur in discontinuous, out-of-phase steps. During the stationary phase, as described above, sodium chloride is transported out of the ascending limb to establish a gradient of 200 mosmol/L, and water diffuses out of the descending limb until descending limb and interstitium have the same osmolarity. During the flow phase, fluid leaves the loop via the distal tubule, and new fluid enters the loop from the proximal tubule (Fig. 20).

Note that the fluid is progressively concentrated as it flows down the descending limb and then is progressively diluted as it flows up the ascending limb. While only a 200 mosmol/L gradient is maintained across the ascending limb at any giving *horizontal level* in the medulla, there exists a much larger osmotic gradient from the top of the medulla to the bottom (312 mosmol/L versus 700 mosmol/L). In other words, the 200 mosmol/L gradient established by active ion transport has been *multiplied* because of the *countercurrent* flow (i.e., flow in opposing directions through the two limbs of a loop) within the loop. It should be emphasized that the active-chloride-transport mechanism within the ascending limb is the essential component of the entire system; without it, the countercurrent flow would have no effect whatsoever on concentrations.

The highest concentration achieved at the tip of the loop depends upon many factors, particularly the length of the loop (the kangaroo rat has extremely long loops) and the strength of the chloride pump. In humans, the value reached is 1400 mosmol/L, which, you will recall, is also the maximal concentration of the excreted urine. But what has this system really accomplished? Certainly, it concentrates the loop fluid to 1400 mosmol/L, but then it immediately redilutes the fluid so that the fluid entering the distal tubule is actually more dilute than the plasma. Where is the *final urine* concentrated and how?

The site of final concentration is in the medullary collecting ducts. Recall that the collecting ducts course through the renal medulla, parallel to the loops of Henle, and are bathed by the interstitial fluid of the medulla. As described above, in the presence of maximal levels of ADH, fluid leaves the cortical collecting tubules isoosmotic to plasma, i.e., at 300 mosmol/L. As this fluid flows through the medullary collecting ducts, it equilibrates with the everincreasing osmolarity of the interstitial fluid. Thus, the real function of the loop countercurrent multiplier system is to

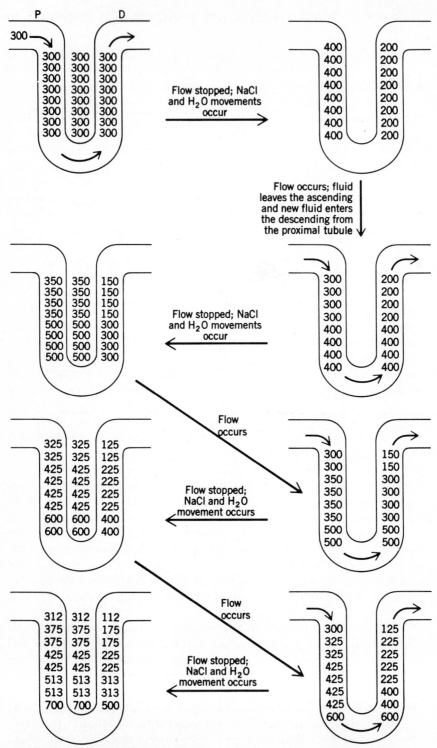

Figure 20 Countercurrent multiplier system in loop of Henle. *(Redrawn from R. F. Pitts, Physiology of the Kidney and Body Fluids, 3d ed., Year Book, Chicago, 1974.)*

concentrate the _medullary interstitium_. Under the influence of ADH, the collecting ducts are highly permeable to water, which diffuses out of the collecting ducts and into the interstitium as a result of the osmotic gradient (Fig. 21). The net result is that the fluid at the end of the collecting duct has equilibrated with the interstitial fluid at the tip of the medulla. In contrast, in the presence of low plasma-ADH concentrations, the collecting ducts become relatively impermeable to water, and the interstitial osmotic gradient is ineffective in inducing water movement out of them.

Because the osmolarity of the urine becomes greater than that of plasma only in the medullary collecting ducts, it is easy to forget that ADH acts not only on this segment but on the late distal tubules and cortical collecting tubules as well. The action on these segments is equally crucial because by permitting the reabsorption there of a large quantity of fluid, it ensures the delivery to the medullary collecting ducts of a volume of isoosmotic fluid small enough for efficient concentrating.

Let us summarize the overall net movement of sodium chloride and water out of the tubules and into the medullary interstitium during formation of a concentrated urine. First, sodium chloride is lost from the ascending limb by active transport of the chloride and passive following by

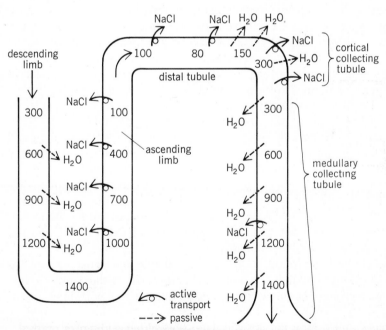

Figure 21 Interactions of loop of Henle and collecting duct in formation of a concentrated urine. As described in the text, this figure is oversimplified in that it assumes active transport by the entire ascending loop and ignores the role of urea. It also ignores the existence of sodium transport by the collecting ducts. (See Chap. 5.)

the sodium.[1] This sodium chloride causes net diffusion of water out of the descending limb and the collecting ducts. In the steady state, this sodium chloride and water entering the medullary interstitium must be taken up by capillaries and carried away. This is, of course, the final step during reabsorption of fluid anywhere in the tubules, and it occurs as a result of the usual hydraulic and oncotic forces acting across the capillary wall.

Countercurrent Exhange: Vasa Recta

There is, however, a unique characteristic of the medullary circulation without which the entire system could not operate, namely, the hairpin-loop anatomy of the medullary vessels (the *vasa recta*), which run parallel to the loops of Henle and medullary collecting ducts (Fig. 5). The problem is this: What would happen to the medullary gradient if the medulla were supplied with ordinary (as opposed to hairpin-loop) capillaries? As plasma having the usual osmolarity of 300 mosmol/L entered the highly concentrated environment of the medulla, there would be massive net diffusion of sodium chloride into the capillaries and of water out of them. Thus, the interstitial gradient would soon be lost. But, with hairpin loops, the sequence of events shown in Fig. 22 occurs. Blood enters the capillary loop at an osmolarity of 300 mosmol/L, and as it flows down the capillary loop deeper and deeper into the medulla, sodium chloride does indeed diffuse into, and water out of, the capillary. However, after the bend in the loop is reached, the blood then flows up the ascending capillary loop, where the process is almost completely reversed. Thus, the capillary loop is acting as a so-called *countercurrent exchanger*, which prevents the gradient from being dissipated. Note that the capillary is, itself, completely passive; i.e., it is not *creating* the medullary gradient, only protecting it. Its passive nature explains why it is called an exchanger; compare its function to that of the loop of Henle, which actively creates the gradient and is, therefore, a multiplier. Finally, it should be noted that the hairpin-loop structure essentially eliminates losses, by *diffusion,* of solute or water from the interstitium. It does not, though, prevent the *bulk flow* of medullary interstitial fluid into the vasa recta secondary to the usual Starling forces. By this bulk-flow process, the net salt and water entering the interstitium from the loops and collecting ducts is carried away, and the steady-state gradient is maintained.

The above description of the countercurrent multiplier system for urinary concentration underestimates the complexity of the overall operation. A major ignored complexity is the fact that the thin portion of the ascending loop of Henle may function differently from the thick portion, specifically that it may not actively transport either sodium or chloride.

---

[1] As described earlier, sodium is also actively reabsorbed from the collecting ducts. This phenomenon helps to reduce the amount of salt lost to the urine. But it has been ignored in our analysis because it is not an important component of the countercurrent system. (See Giebisch and Windhager, 1973, in Suggested Readings for Chap. 6.)

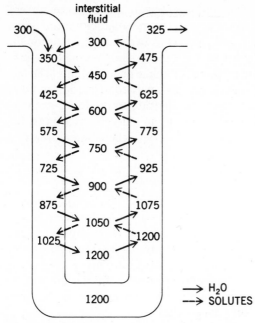

Figure 22 Vasa recta as countercurrent exchangers. *(Redrawn from R. F. Pitts, Physiology of the Kidney and Body Fluids, 3d ed., Year Book, Chicago, 1974.)*

(The evidence for or against this is presently not decisive.) Should such prove to be the case, what is the mechanism by which sodium chloride leaves the thin portion of the ascending limb? (That sodium chloride *does* move from the lumen of this thin portion into the interstitium is well proven—the question at hand here deals only with what the force is that causes it to move.) One hypothesis explains this movement by invoking a special role for urea, and the interested reader should consult the article by Kokko cited in the Suggested Readings for this chapter. Whether or not urea performs this special role, it is definitely involved in another way in the urine concentrating mechanism, specifically in determining maximal concentrating ability. Indeed, of the 1400 mosmol in a liter of urine, almost half of this is urea, and much of the medullary gradient is made up of urea. (Other ions, too, play at least minor roles.) However, we have chosen not to discuss these other complex variables but to focus attention on the absolutely essential factors, namely, the interactions between sodium chloride and water movements in the loops of Henle, collecting ducts, and vasa recta.

A point of considerable clinical importance is that inability to achieve maximal urinary concentration occurs early in any renal disease because of interference with the establishment of the medullary gradient. Any significant change in renal structure, particularly in the medulla, can upset the intricate geometric relationships required for maximal countercurrent functioning. A change in renal blood flow to the medulla, either too much or too little, will reduce the gradient by carrying away too much or too little water and/or solute. Destruction of the loops will also reduce the gradient, as will decreased chloride pumping by the ascending limb. The latter may be caused by tubular disease or by a marked reduction in GFR and, thereby, a reduction in the supply of chloride to the loop. Another important factor is flow rate through the loop; any large increase (as, for exan.ple, in osmotic diuresis) literally "washes out" the gradient, thereby preventing concentration of the final urine.

Finally, it should be emphasized that, although the entire discussion of renal concentrating ability has been in terms of urine osmolarity, the usual clinical measurement of urine "concentration" is *specific gravity*. The determination of specific gravity requires only a hydrometer and is easy and cheap to perform. However, specific gravity is really a measure of urine density, not of concentration. Frequently, the two correlate well, but under certain circumstances they can be quite divergent, since specific gravity is influenced by the nature as well as by the number of solute particles. For example, protein in the urine causes the specific gravity to be increased with little change in osmolarity.

SUMMARY

Figure 23 summarizes the previously described changes in volume and osmolarity of the tubular fluid as it flows along the nephron.

1 Approximately 65 percent of the filtered water and sodium chloride are reabsorbed in the proximal tubule, but the fluid remains isoosmotic.

2 In the loop, water is reabsorbed from the descending limb, but much more sodium chloride is reabsorbed from the ascending limb so that hypoosmotic fluid enters the distal tubule.

3 Fluid remains hypoosmotic in the early distal tubule with little or no water reabsorption occurring.

4 Only from the late distal tubules on does the presence or absence of ADH matter. With essentially no ADH, very little water is reabsorbed from the late distal tubules and collecting ducts. Consequently, a large volume of dilute urine is formed.

5 With maximal ADH, water reabsorption is high in the late distal tubules and collecting ducts. By the end of the cortical portions of the collecting duct system (the cortical collecting tubules), the fluid has once more become isoosmotic. Almost all the remaining water is reabsorbed in the medullary collecting ducts, and a tiny volume of highly concentrated urine is formed. Because of the focus on sodium chloride in this chapter, the reader may be surprised to discover that a maximally concentrated urine (1400 mosmol/L) may, under certain conditions, contain virtually no

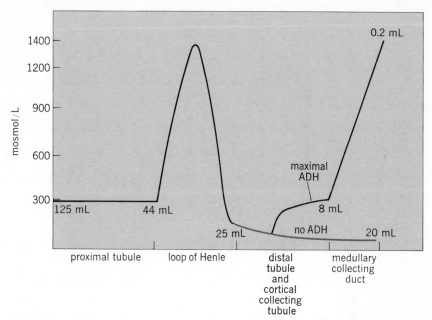

Figure 23 Changes in volume and osmolarity of the tubular fluid as it flows along the nephron.

sodium chloride; the solute may be urea, creatinine, uric acid, potassium, etc. In other words, although sodium chloride *in the medullary interstitium* is the essential requirement for pulling water out of the collecting ducts and concentrating the urine, there need be no sodium chloride in the final urine, itself.

Several other points of great importance should be reemphasized: (1) Excretion of large quantities of sodium *always* results in the excretion of large quantitites of water. This follows from the passive nature of water reabsorption since water can be reabsorbed only if sodium is reabsorbed first. As we shall see, this relationship has considerable importance for the regulation of extracellular volume. (2) In contrast, large quantities of water can be excreted even though the urine is virtually free of sodium since a decreased ADH will increase water excretion without altering sodium transport significantly. This process we shall find crucial for the renal regulation of extracellular osmolarity.

Given the basic renal processes for handling sodium, chloride, and water, we now turn to the mechanisms by which they are controlled so as to homeostatically regulate salt and water balance.

Study questions: **21** to **27**

Chapter 7

Control of Sodium and Water Excretion: Regulation of Extracellular Volume and Osmolarity

OBJECTIVES

The student understands the renal regulation of extracellular volume and osmolarity.

1 States the formula relating filtration, reabsorption, and excretion of sodium
2 Describes the nature and locations of receptors in sodium-regulating reflexes
3 Lists the efferent inputs controlling GFR and how these inputs change as a result of changes in sodium balance or fluid volumes
4 Defines glomerulotubular balance and describes its significance
5 States the origin of aldosterone, its sites of action, and its effects
6 Lists the factors controlling aldosterone secretion and states which is most important
7 Lists the four major factors controlling renin secretion
8 Defines natriuretic hormone
9 Describes how peritubular-capillary dynamics (physical factors) influence sodium reabsorption; states how changes in filtration fraction influence sodium reabsorption; predicts the changes in physical factors

which occur with changes in sodium or fluid balance and how they alter sodium and water reabsorption

10 Defines redistribution of blood flow and states how it might influence sodium and water excretion

11 States all direct and indirect effects of catecholamines and angiotensin on sodium reabsorption

12 Lists all the actions of angiotensin which increase arterial blood pressure

13 Distinguishes between primary and secondary hyperaldosteronism; describes the hormonal changes in each and the presence or absence of "escape"

14 Describes the origin of ADH and the reflex controls of its secretion; defines diabetes insipidus

15 Distinguishes between the reflex changes which occur when an individual has suffered fluid loss because of diarrhea as opposed to a pure water loss, i.e., solute-water loss as opposed to pure-water loss

16 Calculates the changes in body-fluid volumes and osmolarity resulting from the excretion of a known volume of urine having a given osmolarity; defines free-water clearance (both positive and negative)

17 Describes the control of thirst

18 Diagrams in flow-sheet form the pathways by which sodium and water excretion are altered in response to sweating, diarrhea, hemorrhage, high- or low-salt diet

Since sodium is freely filterable at the glomerulus and actively reabsorbed but not secreted by the tubules, the amount of sodium excreted in the final urine represents the results of two processes, glomerular filtration and tubular reabsorption:

$$\text{Sodium excretion} = \text{sodium filtered} - \text{sodium reabsorbed}$$
$$= (\text{GFR} \times P_{\text{Na}}) - \text{sodium reabsorbed}$$

It is possible, therefore, to adjust sodium excretion by controlling any of these three variables (Fig. 24). In fact, P_{Na} generally shows little variation, and the control of GFR and sodium reabsorption predominate. For example, what happens if the quantity of filtered sodium increases as a result of a higher GFR but the rate of reabsorption remains constant? Clearly, sodium excretion increases. The same final result could be achieved by lowering sodium reabsorption while the GFR remains constant. Finally, sodium excretion could be raised greatly by elevating the GFR and simultaneously reducing reabsorption. Conversely, sodium excretion could be decreased below normal levels by lowering the GFR or by raising sodium reabsorption, or by both.

The reflex pathways by which changes in total body sodium balance lead to changes in GFR and sodium reabsorption include: (1) "volume"

FILTERED   REABSORBED   EXCRETED
Na$^+$ Na$^+$ Na$^+$

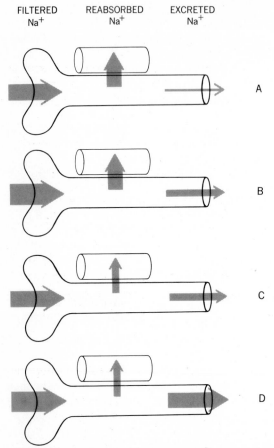

Figure 24   Sodium excretion is increased by increasing the GFR (B), by decreasing reabsorption (C), or by a combination of both (D). The arrows indicate relative magnitudes of filtration, reabsorption, and excretion. *(From A. J. Vander et al., Human Physiology, © 1970 by McGraw-Hill, Inc. Used with permission of McGraw-Hill Book Company.)*

receptors and the afferent pathways leading from them to the central nervous system and endocrine glands; (2) efferent neural and hormonal pathways to the kidneys; and (3) renal effector sites, i.e., the renal arterioles and tubules.

The first component of the reflexes, the so-called volume receptors, offers certain theoretical difficulties. In most physiological control mechanisms, reflexes regulating the magnitude of any given variable (glucose, P_{O_2}, etc.) are initiated by receptors sensitive to changes in that variable. One might, therefore, have expected that reflexes which regulate sodium balance would involve sodium receptors. As we shall see, there are sodium-sensitive receptors in various locations of the body (notably in the adrenal cortex, macula densa of the renal tubules, and brain), but they are not the most important receptors in sodium-controlling reflexes. However, this should not really be too surprising, since what is being held constant by these reflexes is not the *concentration* of sodium in the body fluids but the *total mass* of sodium in the body. Therefore, one must look for some other variable which correlates closely with total body sodium and which might constitute the critical signal. As shown in the following examples, the ideal candidate is the volume of extracellular fluid.

What happens when a person ingests a liter of isotonic sodium chloride, i.e., a solution of salt with exactly the same osmolarity as the body fluids? It is absorbed from the gastrointestinal tract into the plasma, from which most of it then enters the interstitial fluid. The important fact is that all the salt and water remain in the extracellular fluid (plasma and interstitial fluid) and none enters the cells. Because of the active sodium pumps in cell membranes, sodium is effectively barred from the cells. The water, too, remains since only the volume and not the osmolarity of the extracellular compartment has been changed; i.e., no osmotic gradient exists to drive the ingested water into cells. Another example: A person ingests 145 mmol of sodium chloride but no water. The salt is distributed in the extracellular fluid but is barred from the cells. The addition of this water-free solute to the extracellular fluid causes extracellular osmolarity to rise above intracellular osmolarity; therefore, water diffuses out of the cells and into the extracellular fluid until the osmolarities are once more equal. The net result is an expansion of extracellular volume and a decrease of intracellular volume.

These examples lead us to the extremely important generalization that the total extracellular-fluid volume depends primarily upon the mass of extracellular sodium, which, in turn, correlates directly with total body sodium, since sodium is effectively barred from cells. (There are considerable amounts of sodium in bone, but this fact does not seriously alter the analysis.) It should now be clear why reflexes which maintain extracellular volume constant simultaneously keep total body sodium constant in normal persons.

Yet how can there be receptors capable of detecting changes in the total extracellular volume? The answer is almost certainly that there are not any and that total extracellular volume per se is not *directly* monitored. What about its component volumes—plasma volume and interstitial volume? Again neither of these is *directly* monitored; instead, the variables monitored in sodium-regulating reflexes are those that are altered as a result of changes in these volumes (Fig. 25)—notably *intravascular* and *intracardiac* pressures. For example, a decrease in plasma volume generally tends to lower the hydraulic pressures within the veins, cardiac chambers, and arteries; these changes are detected by baroreceptors within those structures, e.g., the carotid sinus, and initiate the re-

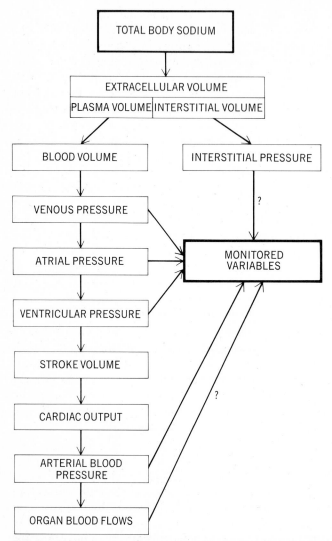

Figure 25 Flow sheet demonstrating the series of derivative variables dependent upon total body sodium. In no case is any block in the sequence totally dependent upon the previous one, for other factors are also involved. The major aim of the figure is to demonstrate how a change in body sodium could result in changes in a group of monitored variables which could be detected by receptors and initiate the responses controlling sodium excretion.

flexes leading to renal sodium retention, which helps restore the plasma volume toward normal. As shown in Fig. 25, other derivatives of extracellular volume which might be detected are organ blood flows and interstitial pressures; however, a role for these variables and others that have been postulated has not been convincingly documented.

To recapitulate, receptors sensitive to sodium (or chloride) do exist and contribute to the regulation of total body sodium, but the major receptors involved in this regulation are those which respond to changes in pressure (or distention) in the cardiovascular system. In the normal person, regulation of these variables results in excellent homeostasis of body sodium and extracellular-fluid volume, since these parameters are all so dependent upon one another. However, as we shall see, disease states can produce striking discrepancies between them with a resulting abnormal expansion of extracellular volume and total body sodium.

Several qualifications should be added to this general scheme. First, this entire description has been in terms of "reflexes," but the fact is, as we shall see, several of the receptors cited are within the kidneys themselves, and no "reflex" input to or output from the kidneys is required in the sequences of events they elicit. Second, the kidneys are influenced directly by changes in the blood perfusing them—for example, by oncotic pressure—so that such nonreflex inputs related to altered sodium balance are also important in determining sodium excretion.

CONTROL OF GFR

We have described the three factors which determine the GFR: glomerular-capillary blood pressure, Bowman's capsule hydraulic pressure, and plasma protein concentration (i.e., plasma oncotic pressure). Anything which alters the magnitude of these factors can be expected to change the GFR. Physiologically, the GFR is controlled primarily by the alteration both of glomerular-capillary pressure and of plasma protein concentration.

Physiological Regulation of Glomerular-Capillary Pressure

(1) A fall in arterial blood pressure decreases filtration rate by lowering glomerular-capillary pressure. Conversely, an increase in arterial blood pressure has just the opposite effect. Recall, however, that, because of renal autoregulation, arterial-pressure changes per se have only small effects on GFR over the usual physiological range. On the other hand, any large decrease in arterial pressure definitely would significantly reduce glomerular-capillary pressure and, thereby, GFR.

(2) A decrease in the diameter of the afferent arterioles, secondary to increased renal sympathetic activity or circulating epinephrine, lowers glomerular-capillary pressure and filtration rate because a larger fraction of the arterial pressure is dissipated in overcoming the increased resistance offered by the narrowed arterioles. These sympathetic pathways, previously described in Chap. 4, play prominent roles in the reflexes which regulate arterial blood pressure, being activated by a lowered

blood pressure and inhibited by an elevated pressure. Let us take a specific example: What changes in renal hemodynamics occur as a result of severe salt and water loss due to diarrhea (Fig. 26)? The decreased plasma volume resulting from salt and water loss prevents adequate venous return, thereby reducing atrial pressure, cardiac output, and arterial blood pressure. These drops in blood pressure are detected by the carotid sinuses and aortic arch, as well as by other baroreceptors in the veins and atria. The information (decreased firing rate of the baroreceptors) is relayed to the medullary cardiovascular centers, which respond by inhibiting parasympathetic outflow to the heart and by stimulating sympathetic outflow to the heart and to arteriolar smooth muscle. The sympathetic stimulation of the renal arterioles (both by the renal nerves and by epinephrine from the adrenal medulla) increases constriction of the renal arterioles. This vasoconstriction increases the resistance to blood flow from the renal artery to the glomerular capillaries, lowering the capillary blood pressure and GFR. By this mechanism, both the amount of sodium filtered and the amount of sodium excreted are reduced, and further loss from the body is prevented. Conversely, an increased GFR can result from greater plasma volume and contribute to increased renal sodium loss, which returns extracellular volume to normal. This analysis is in terms of a logical stimulus for GFR control, namely, changes in blood pressure, but the sympathetic outflow to the kidneys can be changed in response to a variety of stimuli, such as pain, fright, and exercise; accordingly, fluid excretion may be altered at least transiently by many situations.

In this and subsequent discussions we emphasize the significance of the sympathetic nervous system as a major efferent pathway for GFR regulation. As noted in Chap. 4, under the conditions of our example, renin secretion would also be stimulated so that increased plasma angiotensin would contribute to renal vasoconstriction. Again, as described in Chap. 4, prostaglandins would partially oppose the actions of both the sympathetic nerves and angiotensin. These additional details should not obscure the basic fact that the sympathetic nervous system is the dominant reflex pathway for controlling GFR.

Physiological Changes in Plasma Protein Concentration

There are frequent situations in which changes in plasma or extracellular volume are associated with changes in plasma protein concentration. In such situations, changes in oncotic pressure may also play an important role in the physiological raising or lowering of GFR. For example, the severe fluid loss of sweating or diarrhea (Fig. 26) will lower the extracellular volume, but at the same time it will concentrate plasma protein. The resulting increase in oncotic pressure will reduce net filtration pressure in

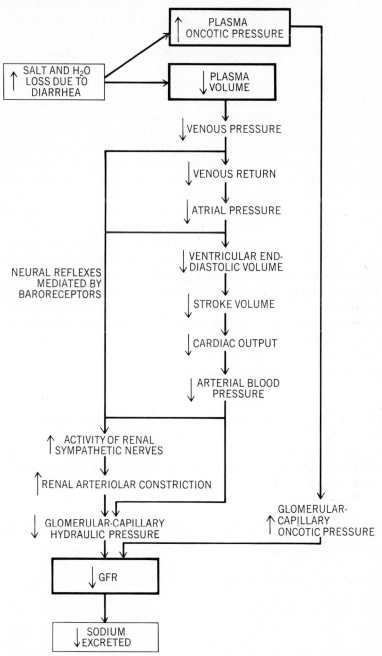

Figure 26 Major pathways by which the GFR is decreased when plasma volume decreases. The baroreceptors which initiate the sympathetic reflex are probably located in large veins and in the walls of the heart, as well as in the carotid sinuses and aortic arch. For clarity, circulating catecholamines and the renin-angiotensin system have not been included in the figure. *(Modified from A. J. Vander et al., Human Physiology, © 1970 by McGraw-Hill, Inc. Used with permission of McGraw-Hill Book Company.)*

the glomeruli and, thereby, GFR. Conversely, a marked increase in salt intake will increase extracellular volume and, at least transiently, lower plasma protein concentration. The result is lowered oncotic pressure and increased GFR.

In each of these examples, the change in arterial plasma protein concentration is in the appropriate direction to reestablish salt balance by decreasing or increasing salt excretion. Is this also true for hemorrhage? The answer is *no*. Hemorrhage per se does not immediately alter plasma protein concentration, since all blood components are lost in *equivalent* proportions. However, the blood loss is followed by a net movement of interstitial fluid into the vascular compartment. This entry of protein-free fluid lowers the plasma protein concentration, which tends to raise GFR—an inappropriate response, since sodium conservation, not increased sodium loss, is the "desired" response to hemorrhage. However, GFR does decrease in response to hemorrhage despite the fact that oncotic pressure is going in the wrong direction. Why? Because decreased arterial pressure and reflexly increased sympathetic outflow to the afferent arterioles cause glomerular-capillary pressure to fall by a larger amount than oncotic pressure falls.[1] This example is presented as a reminder of the fact that renal responses to any given situation represent the algebraic sum of multiple inputs.

CONTROL OF TUBULAR SODIUM REABSORPTION

Present evidence indicates that, so far as long-term regulation of sodium excretion is concerned, the control of tubular sodium reabsorption is probably more important than that of GFR (even though, as we shall see, the former is somewhat dependent on the latter). For example, patients with chronic marked reductions of GFR usually maintain normal sodium excretion by decreasing tubular sodium reabsorption.

Glomerulotubular Balance

One reason for the lesser importance of changes in the filtered load of sodium is the fact that the absolute reabsorption of fluid in the proximal tubules, and probably the loops of Henle and distal tubules as well, varies directly with glomerular filtration rate. This phenomenon is known as *glomerulotubular balance*. For example, if GFR is experimentally decreased by 25 percent (by tightening a clamp around the renal artery), the absolute rate of proximal fluid reabsorption is observed to decrease by almost the same percentage. Another way of saying this is that the percentage of the filtrate reabsorbed proximally remains approximately con-

---

[1]Deen et al., 1974 (Suggested Readings) describe another factor controlling glomerular oncotic pressure.

stant (at 65 percent). The mechanisms responsible for automatically adjusting tubular reabsorption to GFR are not clear.[1] It is certain, however, that they are completely intrarenal; i.e., glomerulotubular balance requires no external neural or hormonal input and can be shown to occur in a completely isolated kidney. The net effect of this phenomenon is to *blunt* the ability of GFR changes per se to produce *large* changes in sodium excretion. However, for several reasons, it is incorrect to assume that, because of glomerulotubular balance, sodium excretion is *completely* unaffected by changes in filtered load. First, even if glomerulotubular balance were perfect, i.e., if the changes in GFR and reabsorption were exactly proportional, the *absolute* amounts of sodium leaving the proximal tubule would still change when GFR changes; this can be seen in the example given in Table 8—even though reabsorption stays fixed at 66.7 percent, the amount of sodium leaving the proximal tubule rises when GFR is increased and falls when GFR is decreased. Second, glomerulotubular balance is not really perfect; i.e., the changes in GFR and reabsorption are not usually exactly proportional. The proper conclusion is that changes in the filtered load of sodium per se do result in changes in sodium excretion, but the changes are greatly mitigated by glomerulotubular balance.

In a sense, glomerulotubular balance is a second line of defense preventing changes in hemodynamics per se from causing large changes in sodium excretion. The first line of defense is GFR autoregulation. In other words, autoregulation prevents GFR from changing too much in direct response to changes in blood pressure, and glomerulotubular balance blunts the sodium-excretion response to whatever GFR change does occur. This allows major responsibility for control of sodium excretion to reside in those factors, to be described next, which act specifically to influence tubular reabsorption of sodium above and beyond any change induced directly by GFR changes. We also see here another analogy between autoregulation and glomerulotubular balance in that both are manifest in their "pure" forms only when the kidneys are manipulated in relative iso-

---

[1]See de Wardener, 1978 (Suggested Readings).

Table 8   Effect of "Perfect" Glomerulotubular Balance on the Mass of Sodium Leaving the Proximal Tubule

GFR, L/min	P_{Na}, mmol/L	Filtered, mmol/min	Reabsorbed proximally (66.7% of filtered), mmol/min	Leaving proximal, mmol/min
0.124	145	18	12	6
0.165	145	24	16	8
0.062	145	9	6	3

lation from the rest of the body, as by altering renal perfusion through the use of renal-artery clamps; in contrast, when GFR is made to change by doing something to the whole animal or person, say by infusing large quantities of isotonic saline, glomerulotubular balance can be overridden by other inputs to the kidney so that the proximal tubule is observed to reabsorb a smaller percentage (in our saline-infusion example) or a larger percentage (in situations like severe hemorrhage) than usual. The same is true for other nephron segments which manifest glomerulotubular balance.

Aldosterone

A major clue to the control of sodium reabsorption was the observation that patients whose adrenal glands are diseased or missing excrete large quantities of sodium in the urine. Indeed, if untreated, they may die because of low blood pressure resulting from depletion of plasma volume. This increased sodium excretion often occurs despite lowered GFR, thus establishing that decreased tubular reabsorption is the factor responsible for the sodium loss. The adrenal influence on sodium reabsorption is mediated by a hormone, *aldosterone,* produced by the *adrenal cortex,* specifically in the cortical area known as the *zona glomerulosa.* (This term is somewhat unfortunate because it sounds like a description of a kidney area rather than of an adrenal zone.)

Aldosterone stimulates sodium reabsorption in the distal tubules and collecting ducts; an action on these distal portions of the nephron is just what one would expect for a fine-tuning input since approximately 90 percent of the filtered sodium has already been reabsorbed (by the proximal tubule and ascending loop of Henle) by the beginning of the distal tubule. The total quantity of sodium reabsorption dependent upon the influence of aldosterone is approximately 2 percent of the total filtered sodium (or, said in another way, 20 percent of the sodium entering the distal tubules). Thus, in the complete absence of aldosterone, one would excrete 2 percent of the filtered sodium; whereas, in the presence of maximal plasma concentrations of aldosterone, virtually no sodium would be excreted. Two percent of the filtered sodium may, at first thought, seem small, but it is actually very large because of the huge volume of glomerular filtrate:

$$\text{Total filtered NaCl/day} = \text{GFR} \times P_{\text{Na}}$$
$$= 180 \text{ L/day} \times 145 \text{ mmol/L}$$
$$= 26,100 \text{ mmol/day}$$

Thus, aldosterone controls the reabsorption of $0.02 \times 26,100$ mmol/day = 522 mmol/day. In terms of sodium chloride, the form in which most sodium is ingested, this amounts to approximately 30 g NaCl per day, an amount considerably more than the average person eats. Therefore, by reflex variation of plasma concentrations of aldosterone between minimal and maximal, the excretion of sodium can be finely adjusted to the intake so that total body sodium and extracellular volume remain constant.

It is interesting that aldosterone also stimulates sodium transport by other epithelia in the body, namely, by sweat and salivary glands and by the intestine. The net effect is the same as that exerted on the kidney—a reduction in the sodium content of the luminal fluid. Thus, aldosterone is an all-purpose stimulator of sodium retention. This hormone, like other steroids, exerts its effect by entering its target cells, combining with cytosolic receptors, migrating into the nucleus in combination with its receptor, and stimulating synthesis of a particular mRNA. Just which protein this mRNA codes for and how the protein, once formed, enhances sodium transport is far from settled. One result of the fact that aldosterone's enhancement of sodium reabsorption requires this time-consuming (at least 45 min) sequence of events is that decreases in sodium excretion which occur within minutes (as, for example, upon standing up) are clearly not due to increased aldosterone.

Control of Aldosterone Secretion   How is aldosterone secretion controlled? At least four distinct inputs to the adrenal gland are recognized at present: (1) plasma sodium concentration, (2) plasma potassium concentration, (3) adrenocorticotropic hormone (ACTH), and (4) angiotensin.

The first two of these inputs are not mediated by nerves or by hormones. Rather, the adrenal cortex responds to the sodium and potassium concentrations of the blood perfusing it or to some adrenal intracellular derivative of these concentrations, such as adrenal-cell sodium concentration. This is one of the true ''sodium'' receptors referred to earlier in this chapter, and the fact that aldosterone secretion is controlled, in part, by plasma sodium concentration makes good sense: Increased plasma sodium → decreased aldosterone secretion → decreased tubular sodium reabsorption → increased sodium excretion → decreased plasma sodium concentration. However, in humans, this is only a minor control of aldosterone secretion—a fact which also makes sense teleologically since plasma sodium *concentration* generally changes very little despite marked changes in extracellular *volume*. (Remember that water movements into or out of body cells tend to keep osmolarity and, thereby, plasma sodium concentration, relatively stable.) The influence of plasma potassium concentration on aldosterone secretion is important and will be described in the section on renal handling of potassium.

ACTH is the hormone from the anterior pituitary which controls secretion of the other major adrenocortical hormone, cortisol. There is no question that when ACTH is secreted in very large amounts, as during physical trauma, it also stimulates aldosterone secretion. However, the relationship of ACTH to sodium homeostasis is not of primary importance.

We are left with our fourth input, angiotensin, as the most important known[1] controller of aldosterone secretion in sodium-regulating reflexes. As described in Chap. 1, the primary determinant of the plasma concentration of angiotensin is the plasma concentration of renin, which is, itself, determined mainly by the rate of renin secretion. Accordingly, control of aldosterone secretion is, in large part, ultimately determined by those factors which regulate renin secretion, to which we now turn. Because the single most important action of the renin-angiotensin system, as regards fluid balance, is its control of aldosterone secretion, description of the control of renin secretion was delayed until now so that the entire flow of events can be better appreciated. (This would be an excellent time to review the basic biochemistry of the renin-angiotensin system and the anatomy of the juxtaglomerular apparatus, both described in Chap. 1.)

Control of Renin Secretion The control of renin secretion is quite complex, since there are at least four major types of inputs, which are, in some ways, strongly interrelated with one another. Indeed, it is proving a very difficult task to untangle them. These four mechanisms are (1) an intrarenal baroreceptor, (2) a tubular sodium (or chloride) receptor in the macula densa, (3) the renal sympathetic nerves, and (4) angiotensin itself.

Intrarenal Baroreceptors The renin-secreting granular cells themselves may act as baroreceptors (i.e., as pressure or distention receptors) monitoring the pressure or vascular volume within the last portions of the afferent arterioles (Fig. 27) and varying their secretion of renin inversely with these parameters. This makes good sense teleologically. For example, consider the response to diarrhea that was described in the section on control of GFR: The pressure at the ends of the afferent arterioles is reduced both because of decreased arterial pressure and because of reflexly increased sympathetic outflow to the arterioles (Fig. 26); the decreased arteriolar pressure would cause increased release of renin from the granular cells (Fig. 28).

Macula Densa Because of the contact between the granular cells and the macula densa (Fig. 27), it is tempting to postulate that the renin-secreting granular cells are controlled, in part, by input from the macula densa concerning the composition of the fluid at the end of the ascending loop of Henle. (Recall that the macula densa is the junction between the loop of Henle and the distal convoluted tubule.) Experimental evidence suggests that this is the case. Specifically, the evidence suggests that renin

---

[1]Several groups of investigators have made a strong case for the existence of important but as yet unidentified aldosterone stimulators in addition to the four mentioned here.

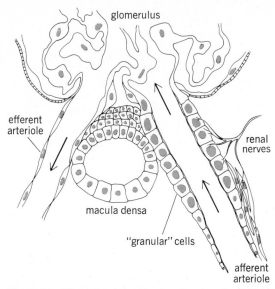

Figure 27 Diagram of glomerulus showing the juxtaglomerular apparatus. The granular cells secrete renin and are also thought to function as baroreceptors. [*Redrawn from J. O. Davis, Am. J. Med.*, **55**:333 (1973).]

secretion is *inversely* related to the mass of sodium chloride flowing into the macula densa.[1] Such a reflex also makes sense teleologically, since it is simply a logical extension of the reflex described for the intrarenal-baroreceptor theory (Fig. 29). Indeed, it should be evident why it has been so difficult to distinguish between the intrarenal-baroreceptor and macula densa theories. At present, it seems likely that both types of receptors exist within the kidney and contribute to the control of renin release. In the situation illustrated by Fig. 29, sodium-chloride load to the macula densa was decreased because of a reduction in GFR. It should be obvious that macula densa sodium-chloride load can also be decreased by increasing proximal and/or loop sodium-chloride reabsorption.

Renal Sympathetic Nerves We have already described one important mechanism by which an increased renal-sympathetic-nerve activity (and

[1]It is hypothesized that the actual signal is not the sodium chloride in the lumen of the macula densa but rather the sodium or chloride concentration of the macula densa cells themselves. In this view, the rate of sodium chloride uptake by the cells is presumably proportional to the mass flowing by them (because of glomerulotubular balance); therefore, the sodium and chloride concentrations of the cell change in proportion to macula densa load, and these changes result in the generation of a chemical signal transmitted to the adjacent granular cells—the signal is inhibitory when the cell concentrations are high and stimulatory when low; whether sodium or chloride is the critical ion is not certain. It must be pointed out that the entire question of the stimulus detected by the macula densa remains very controversial. Indeed, at least one investigator has postulated precisely the reverse of the entire hypothesis just described. (See Davis, 1973, Suggested Readings for Chap. 7, for a review of this field.)

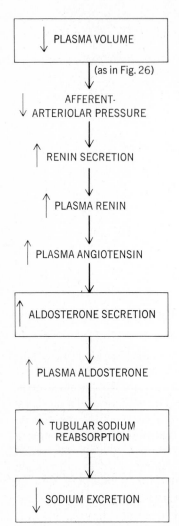

Figure 28 Intrarenal baroreceptor pathway for control of renin release and sodium excretion via changes in aldosterone.

increased circulating epinephrine) stimulates renin secretion, namely, by causing constriction of the afferent arterioles. This stimulates the intrarenal baroreceptor by reducing the hydrostatic pressure at the end of the afferent arteriole, and it also stimulates the macula densa receptor by reducing GFR and, thereby, the sodium load leaving the loop of Henle. In this manner, the renal sympathetic nerves clearly play an important *indirect* role in controlling renin secretion. In addition, sympathetic neurons end in the immediate vicinity of the granular cells (Fig. 27), and these neurons exert a *direct* stimulatory effect on renin secretion via beta-

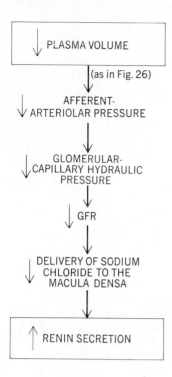

Figure 29 Macula densa pathway for control of renin release. Macula densa sodium load would probably also be reduced because of increased proximal and loop sodium reabsorption, as will be described later in this chapter.

adrenergic receptors on the granular cells. Figure 30 summarizes the interactions of the intrarenal receptors and sympathetic nervous system.

   Angiotensin   Angiotensin exerts a direct inhibitory effect on renin secretion by the granular cells. This is an example of a negative-feedback loop in which a hormone inhibits the secretion of its own stimulating substance, analogous to the inhibition of ACTH secretion by cortisol or to inhibition of TSH secretion by thyroxin. By this mechanism, angiotensin exerts a dampening effect upon its own rate of production.

   Other Inputs Controlling Renin Release   There are many inputs other than the four just described which have been shown to be capable of altering renin release; these include, among others, ADH, potassium, and calcium (all of which can inhibit renin release). The physiological significance of these pathways is mainly that they provide additional loops in the feedback mechanisms integrating the metabolism of sodium with that of water and other ions. Under most circumstances, they are only of minor importance, but this may not be true in clinical situations characterized by a large excess or deficit of any of them.[1] Of particular interest is

[1]For further information, consult Davis, 1973, and Laragh and Sealey, 1973, in Suggested Readings for Chap. 7.

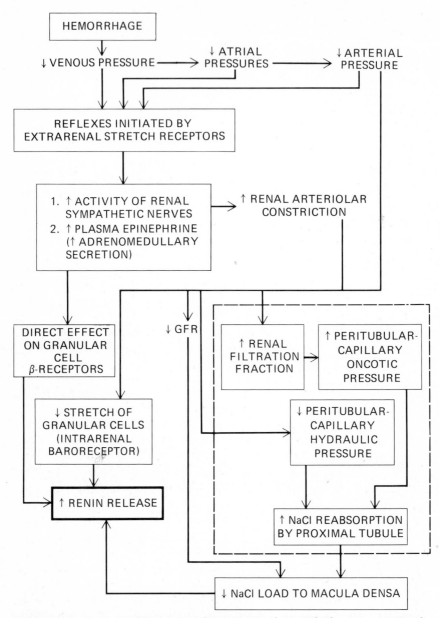

Figure 30   Interactions of the intrarenal receptors and sympathetic nervous system in stimulation of renin release during hemorrhage. This is an amalgamation of the pathways already shown in Figs. 28 and 29, with the addition of the direct action of the sympathetic nervous system on the JG apparatus. The way in which proximal sodium reabsorption might be increased (enclosed by the dashed box) is described later in this chapter.

yet another potential input—renal prostaglandins. In Chap. 4, it was pointed out that angiotensin stimulates the release of prostaglandins, but it also seems that prostaglandins may influence renin secretion (in both inhibitory and stimulatory ways). However, we are not yet certain as to the precise significance of this pathway.

Factors Other Than Aldosterone which Influence Tubular Reabsorption of Sodium

Despite its great importance in the regulation of tubular reabsorption of sodium, aldosterone is not the only factor which does so in response to alterations in body-sodium balance. Identification of these other factors has been easily the most investigated subject in renal physiology during the past decade, but we are still left with great uncertainty concerning the quantitative significance of the many such factors which have been uncovered. Accordingly, one can presently do little more than describe briefly each of the major candidates.

Natriuretic Hormone   The evidence for the existence of a *natriuretic,* or salt-losing, hormone is highly controversial but seems to be growing more solid. It suggests that such a hormone is released when extracellular volume is expanded and that it acts upon the collecting ducts to inhibit sodium reabsorption.[1] Conversely, one would presume that its basal secretion would be inhibited when extracellular volume is contracted, with the result that sodium reabsorption by the collecting ducts is enhanced. The site of production of this hypothesized natriuretic hormone is not known nor are the pathways which might control it.

Intrarenal Physical Factors: Interstitial Hydraulic Pressure   A factor which can strongly influence net fluid reabsorption is the hydraulic pressure in the renal intercellular compartment (interstitium). Recall from the previous chapter that although interstitial hydraulic pressure is one of the minor forces favoring the last step in fluid reabsorption—movement into the peritubular capillaries—it also constitutes an important force simultaneously driving fluid back into the tubular lumen across the tight junctions between cells. This back-leakage, of course, reduces *net* tubular fluid reabsorption, i.e., "short circuits" some of the reabsorption achieved by the forces moving sodium, chloride, and water out of the lumen into the interstitium. The important generalization then is:

---

[1] A fascinating recent finding is consistent with the possibility that, under certain circumstances, the collecting duct may actually *add* sodium to the urine, perhaps stimulated to do so by natriuretic hormone. The existence of such sodium "secretion" would certainly play havoc with conventional theory about renal sodium handling, but other interpretations of the data are possible.

Whenever interstitial hydraulic pressure is elevated, there is a tendency for overall fluid reabsorption to be decreased (because of increased back-leakage);[1] conversely, a decrease in interstitial hydraulic pressure favors fluid reabsorption (because back-leakage is diminished).

The factors which are most important in setting the steady-state interstitial hydraulic pressure in the kidneys are really the same as in any other location in the body—the intracapillary hydraulic and oncotic pressures—since these are the dominant forces determining the steady-state volume of fluid in the interstitium. An increased hydraulic pressure inside the capillary tends to raise interstitial hydraulic pressure by causing fluid to accumulate in the interstitium; a decrease in plasma oncotic pressure does precisely the same. Therefore, via its effects on interstitial hydraulic pressure and back-leakage into the tubular lumen, increased hydraulic pressure in the peritubular capillaries reduces tubular fluid reabsorption. Conversely, decreased peritubular-capillary hydraulic pressure facilitates reabsorption. An increased oncotic pressure in peritubular capillaries also facilitates reabsorption, whereas a decreased oncotic pressure reduces reabsorption. Thus, earlier in this chapter we saw that changes in *glomerular-capillary* hydraulic and oncotic pressures were controlled so as to regulate GFR and, thereby, sodium excretion; now we see that analogous changes in the *peritubular-capillary* hydraulic and oncotic pressures regulate sodium reabsorption and, thereby, sodium excretion.

Teleologically, it makes good sense that such changes in these intrarenal physical factors regulate sodium balance and extracellular volume by altering sodium reabsorption. Volume depletion (as in our example of diarrhea) causes decreased peritubular-capillary hydraulic pressure (just as it does decreased glomerular-capillary hydraulic pressure) because of reduced arterial pressure and reflex renal vasoconstriction (Fig. 31). The effect of the reduced pressure is to enhance sodium reabsorption. The sodium depletion also causes concentration of plasma protein, and this increased oncotic pressure also enhances tubular sodium reabsorption, just as it reduces GFR.

In the last example above, the change in peritubular-capillary oncotic pressure simply reflects a change in systemic plasma oncotic pressure. Now, we introduce a new but predictable fact: Peritubular-capillary oncotic pressure can be changed independently of any changes in systemic oncotic pressure. The information needed to understand this phenomenon has already been given: Peritubular-capillary oncotic pressure *always* differs from systemic oncotic pressure, since the plasma proteins are concentrated by loss of protein-free filtrate during passage through the

---

[1]This is true not only for sodium, chloride, and water but for almost all solutes reabsorbed proximally, the major site of influence by interstitial hydraulic pressure, since the back-leakage involves bulk flow of all interstitial contents.

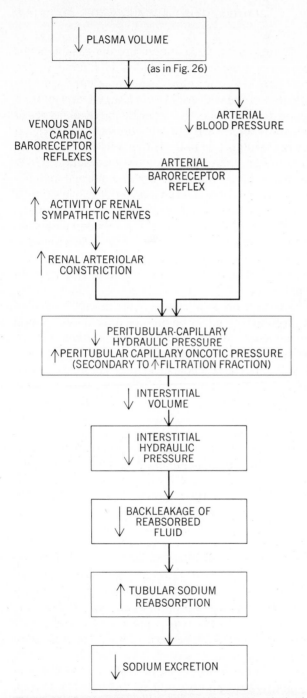

Figure 31 Pathway by which changes in intrarenal physical factors are elicited by changes in plasma volume. Compare this to Fig. 26, the figure for GFR control; clearly the same inputs that tend to lower GFR also tend to increase sodium reabsorption. As with Fig. 26, for simplicity, circulating catecholamines and the renin-angiotensin system have not been included.

glomerular capillaries. The degree of oncotic-pressure increase depends upon the fraction of the renal plasma flow which is filtered at the glomerulus; this *filtration fraction* is not always the same but varies depending upon the distribution of renal arteriolar constriction. Recall from Chap. 4 that reflex vasoconstriction mediated either by the renal nerves or by circulating agents generally affects not only the afferent arterioles but the efferent as well. The net result is that both GFR and RPF decrease but the latter more than the former; therefore, the filtration fraction, GFR/RPF, increases. Accordingly, there occurs a larger-than-normal increase in peritubular-capillary oncotic pressure, and an increased reabsorption of sodium. Conversely, reflexly induced renal vasodilation (as might occur after increased ingestion of salt and water) would be associated with a decreased filtration fraction, a smaller-than-normal rise in peritubular-capillary oncotic pressure, and less sodium reabsorption. Thus, filtration fraction, by altering peritubular-capillary oncotic pressure, is a determinant of sodium reabsorption.

Just how important are these physical factors in the normal control of sodium and water reabsorption? As might be predicted from information given in Chap. 6, their influence is seen mainly in the proximal tubule, since only this nephron segment has tight junctions leaky enough to permit much back-leakage of fluid. There seems little question that when alterations in fluid balance are very large (as, for example, during severe hemorrhage), proximal reabsorption does change mainly because of the large alterations in the physical factors we have been discussing. Whether significant changes in proximal reabsorption occur in response to more modest alterations in fluid balance (as might result, for example, from eating a diet very low or very high in sodium chloride) is still not known for certain.

Redistribution of Blood Flow   Another potential mechanism for altering sodium excretion is *redistribution of blood flow*. It has been hypothesized that certain nephrons may have less capacity to reabsorb sodium than others. Were this true, then at any given total GFR, the relative amounts of fluid filtered by the two different nephron populations would be an important determinant of sodium excretion. Specifically, a redistribution of GFRs to the "high-reabsorption" nephrons, secondary, say, to altered sympathetic input to the two populations, would be associated with decreased sodium excretion because of the greater capacity of these nephrons to reabsorb sodium. Moreover, one can also imagine a redistribution of RPF out of proportion to that of GFR so that filtration fraction and, thereby, fluid reabsorption, could be enhanced in certain nephrons with no change in total renal RPF. Despite the attractiveness of these theories, the evidence in favor of them has not yet been very convincing.

Direct Tubular Effects of Catecholamines   Preceding sections have detailed how the renal sympathetic nerves and circulating epinephrine can influence sodium reabsorption by altering intrarenal physical factors and the secretion of renin. In this section, we now emphasize that these inputs also stimulate sodium reabsorption by a direct action on the tubular cells themselves. (There are numerous neuron terminals adjacent to the tubular cells.) Just which tubular segments are most affected by this direct input (which obviously has the same adaptive significance as the indirect results of altered sympathetic activity) is not yet certain.

Direct Tubular Effects of Angiotensin   This story reads almost identically to the previous paragraph. Angiotensin enhances sodium reabsorption indirectly both through its stimulation of aldosterone and its effects on intrarenal physical factors. (Recall that angiotensin constricts renal arterioles and raises filtration fraction.) In addition, it seems to act directly on the renal cells themselves to stimulate sodium reabsorption.[1] Again, as is the case with the catecholamines, the nephron segments involved have not yet been identified.

We have been chewing at the effects of angiotensin in small bites throughout this book, and this seems an appropriate place to digest them as well as to gulp down those remaining. The fact is that angiotensin exerts a bewildering array of effects on many bodily sites, but the common denominator of those with which we are concerned is that they all favor salt retention and elevation of arterial blood pressure. Figure 32 summarizes these, adding the facts, not previously mentioned, that angiotensin stimulates ADH secretion and thirst and facilitates the activity of the sympathetic nervous system. It is crucial to recognize that when renin secretion is elevated in response to physiological stimuli, such as sodium deprivation, all the effects of angiotensin shown in Fig. 32 serve to minimize fluid depletion and to prevent blood pressure from falling below normal. In contrast, when a *primary* increase in renin secretion occurs due to disease (as in renal artery stenosis, for example), these effects will tend to elevate the blood pressure above normal.

Other Known Humoral Agents   Cortisol, estrogen, growth hormone, and insulin are all known to enhance sodium reabsorption, whereas glucagon, progesterone, and parathyroid hormone all decrease it. It is almost certain that when any of these hormones is elevated (as, for example, estrogen during pregnancy), it will exert a significant influence on sodium reabsorption and, thereby, excretion. However, there is no reason to be-

---

[1]A source of considerable potential confusion is the fact that angiotensin, when present in extremely high ("pharmacological") amounts, inhibits sodium reabsorption rather than stimulating it.

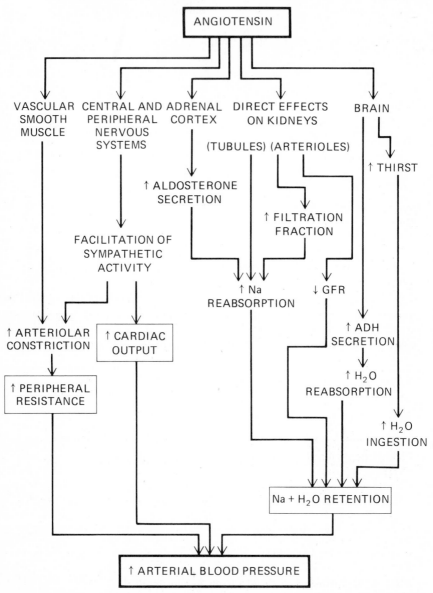

Figure 32 Summary of those angiotensin-mediated actions which facilitate fluid retention and elevate the arterial blood pressure. The arrow connecting "Na and H_2O retention" to "arterial blood pressure" is a shortcut for the sake of simplicity—of course, fluid retention influences arterial blood pressure only by altering cardiac output and peripheral resistance. The effects shown in this figure have all been documented for angiotensin II; some may also be exerted by angiotensin III.

lieve that any of them, unlike the factors described previously, are reflexly controlled specifically so as to homeostatically regulate sodium balance.

Also of great interest is the possible role played by intrarenal humoral systems, particularly the prostaglandins and the kinins. These agents are known to be able to reduce sodium reabsorption, perhaps by altering intrarenal physical factors (as we have seen, they are potent vasodilators) or by direct actions on the tubular cells. Their concentrations are also known to change with alterations of sodium balance, but there is still too little evidence to integrate them with any assurance into the overall picture of renal sodium regulation.

SUMMARY OF THE CONTROL OF SODIUM EXCRETION

The control of sodium excretion depends upon the control of two variables of renal function, the GFR and the rate of sodium reabsorption (Table 9). The latter is controlled by the renin-angiotensin-aldosterone hormone system, the sympathetic nervous system, and several other less well defined factors. The last category probably includes changes in intrarenal hydraulic and oncotic pressures (the so-called physical factors), a natriuretic (or salt-losing) hormone, and, possibly, the distribution of blood flow within the kidney. The renal sympathetic nerves play a prominent role in each of the following: control of aldosterone via renin-angiotensin, determination of intrarenal physical factors, the reabsorptive

Table 9 Changes in These Factors Regulate Sodium Excretion in Response to Changes in Extracellular Volume

Filtration of sodium
  *GFR
  *Plasma sodium concentration (of minor importance except in severe disorders)

Tubular reabsorption of sodium
  *GFR
  *Aldosterone
  *Intrarenal "physical factors"
  *Renal nerves and circulating epinephrine (direct tubular effects)
  Natriuretic hormone
  Angiotensin (direct tubular effects)
  Distribution of GFRs to different nephrons

*Asterisks denote factors for whose participation the evidence is very strong. Roles for the others are likely but have not been conclusively documented. Not listed in the table are factors whose roles are even more speculative (the prostaglandins and kinins, for example) and factors which can influence sodium excretion but which are probably not homeostatically controlled primarily for that "purpose."

activity of the tubular cells themselves, and the control of GFR. Yet because of the many other known (and unknown) factors involved, a transplanted and, therefore, denervated kidney maintains sodium homeostasis quite well.

The reflexes which control both GFR and sodium reabsorption are essentially blood-pressure-regulating reflexes, since they are probably most frequently initiated by changes in arterial or venous pressure. This is fitting, since cardiovascular function depends upon an adequate plasma volume, which, as a component of the extracellular-fluid volume, normally reflects the mass of sodium in the body. In normal persons, these regulatory mechanisms are so precise that sodium balance does not vary by more than 2 percent despite marked changes in dietary intake or losses due to sweating, vomiting, diarrhea, hemorrhage, or burns.

In several types of disease, however, sodium balance becomes deranged by the failure of the kidneys to excrete sodium normally. Sodium excretion may fall virtually to zero and remain there despite continued sodium ingestion, and the patient retains large quantities of sodium and water within the body, leading to abnormal expansion of extracellular fluid and formation of edema. An important example of this phenomenon is congestive heart failure. A patient with a failing heart (i.e., a heart whose contractility is too low to maintain the cardiac output required for the body's metabolic requirements) usually manifests decreased GFR and increased activity of the renin-angiotensin-aldosterone system. In addition, renal filtration fraction is almost always increased—a situation that causes increased oncotic pressure in the peritubular capillaries. All these, and perhaps other sodium-retaining factors, contribute to the almost complete reabsorption of sodium. The net result is expansion of plasma volume, increased capillary pressure, and filtration of fluid into the interstitial space (edema).

Why do these sodium-retaining reflexes continue to be elicited despite the fact that the person is in markedly positive and progressively increasing sodium balance? The answer stems from the fact, described earlier, that total extracellular volume itself is not directly monitored. In the normal person there is no discrepancy between changes in total extracellular volume and total body sodium, on the one hand, and plasma volume, cardiovascular pressures, and cardiac output, on the other. Thus, a reflex triggered by a change in these latter derivative functions will end up homeostatically regulating body sodium and extracellular volume. In contrast, because of his or her failing heart, there is a discontinuity between these two groups of variables; i.e., the patient has an inadequate cardiac output despite an increased extracellular volume. This reduced cardiac output initiates, most likely via arterial baroreceptors (which reduce their firing rates because of the decrease in mean and pulsatile arterial pressure),[1] sodium-retaining reflexes just as would occur in a normal person whose cardiac output had been reduced due to hemorrhage or severe diarrhea.

There are several other conditions, specifically the liver disease cirrhosis and the kidney syndrome nephrosis, that tend to produce sodium retention of this kind. They, too, are characterized by persistent sodium-retaining reflexes (decreased GFR, increased aldosterone, etc.) despite progressive overexpansion of extracellular fluid and formation of edema, as in congestive heart failure. All these edematous conditions, including congestive heart failure, are sometimes called diseases of *secondary hyperaldosteronism* because they are usually associated with increased secretion of aldosterone *secondary* to increased renin, which in turn is due to the inappropriate reflexes just described. At one time it was thought that the elevated aldosterone was sufficient in itself to cause progressive accumulation of sodium. It is now recognized that such is not the case and that one or more of the other factors which influence sodium excretion must also be operating to maintain the retention. This is nicely illustrated by the difference in sodium handling between *primary hyperaldosteronism* and the diseases of secondary hyperaldosteronism. Primary hyperaldosteronism is characterized by persistent oversecretion of aldosterone due to a primary adrenal defect, usually an aldosterone-producing tumor. Because of the increased aldosterone, sodium retention does occur *initially,* but after a few days, there occurs an *escape* from the effects of aldosterone, i.e., a return to normal sodium excretion despite the continued presence of increased aldosterone. (After balance is reestablished, a persistent, small, positive sodium balance does remain.) What has happened is that the initial sodium retention causes expansion of extracellular volume and total body sodium, which then initiates sodium-losing reflexes via changes in GFR and the factors other than aldosterone which control sodium reabsorption. In other words, persistent, progressive sodium retention cannot be induced by an abnormality in only one of the factors controlling sodium excretion, since reflexes will rapidly be induced whereby opposing changes in the other factors will restore normal sodium excretion. Only when essentially all inputs are altering sodium excretion, either appropriately, as in sodium depletion, or inappropriately, as in the diseases of secondary hyperaldosteronism with edema, will sodium excretion remain continuously near zero; in these latter diseases, "escape" does not occur from the effects of persistently elevated aldosterone.

---

[1]In addition, baroreceptors in the great veins and cardiac chambers appear to be damaged by (or adapted to) the engorgement occurring in these locations and manifest decreased rates of firing despite the marked degree of distention.

ADH SECRETION AND EXTRACELLULAR VOLUME

Although we have spoken of extracellular-volume regulation only in terms of the control of sodium excretion, it is clear that, to be most effective in altering extracellular volume, the changes in sodium excretion must be accompanied by equivalent changes in water excretion. We have already pointed out that the ability of water to follow when sodium is reabsorbed depends upon ADH. Accordingly, a decreased extracellular volume must reflexly call forth increased ADH production as well as increased aldosterone secretion. What is the nature of this reflex? ADH is an octapeptide produced by a discrete group of hypothalamic neurons whose cell bodies are located in the supraoptic and paraventricular nuclei and whose axons terminate in the posterior pituitary, from which ADH is released into the blood. These hypothalamic cells receive input from several vascular baroreceptors, particularly a group located in the left atrium (Fig. 33). The baroreceptors are stimulated by increased atrial blood pressure, and the impulses resulting from this stimulation are transmitted via afferent nerves and ascending pathways to the hypothalamus, where they inhibit the ADH-producing cells. Conversely, decreased atrial pressure causes less firing by the baroreceptors and a resulting stimulation of ADH synthesis and release (Fig. 34). The adaptive value of this baroreceptor reflex should require no comment.

As shown in Fig. 32, angiotensin also stimulates ADH release, just as it does aldosterone secretion. Thus, the renin-angiotensin system may play a role in enhancing water reabsorption (via ADH) as it does sodium (via aldosterone), but the quantitative importance of this pathway is almost certainly less than that of the atrial baroreceptor reflex for ADH just described.

ADH AND THE RENAL REGULATION OF EXTRACELLULAR OSMOLARITY

We turn now to the renal compensation for pure-water losses or gains, e.g., the situation in which a person drinks 2 L of water, but no change in the total bodily salt content occurs. Only the total water changes. The most efficient compensatory mechanism is for the kidneys to excrete the excess water without altering its usual excretion of salt, and this is precisely what they do. ADH secretion is reflexly inhibited, as will be described below, water permeability of the more distal segments of the nephron becomes very low, sodium reabsorption proceeds normally but water is unable to follow, and a large volume of extremely dilute urine is excreted. In this manner, the excess pure water is eliminated. Conversely, when a pure-water deficit occurs, ADH secretion is reflexly stimulated, water permeability of these segments is increased, water

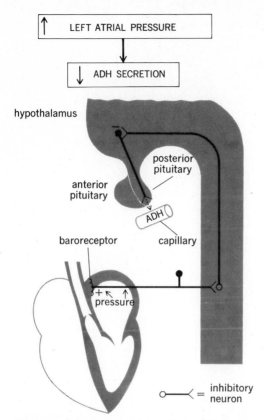

Figure 33 Major pathway by which ADH secretion is decreased when plasma volume is increased. The greater plasma volume raises left atrial pressure, which stimulates the atrial baroreceptors and inhibits ADH secretion. *(From A. J. Vander et al., Human Physiology, © 1970 by McGraw-Hill, Inc. Used with permission of McGraw-Hill Book Company.)*

reabsorption occurs at a maximal rate, the final urine volume becomes extremely small, and its osmolarity is considerably greater than that of the plasma. By this means, relatively less of the filtered water than solute is excreted—which is equivalent to adding pure water to the body—and the pure water deficit is compensated.

The renal contribution to alterations in body-fluid osmolarity is quantifiable through use of a term known as *free-water clearance,* abbreviated C_{H_2O}. Note immediately that the term is not *water* clearance, which would denote, by conventional clearance terminology, the volume of water removed from the plasma per unit time. Instead, free-water clearance is not really a true clearance at all but denotes the volume of *pure water* which would have to be removed from, or added to, the urine to make it isoosmotic to plasma. Let us take as an example the excretion of 1 L of urine

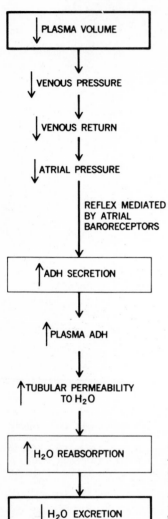

Figure 34 Major pathway by which ADH secretion is increased when plasma volume decreases. This figure is merely the converse of Fig. 33 *(From A. J. Vander et al., Human Physiology,* © *1970 by McGraw-Hill, Inc. Used with permission of McGraw-Hill Book Company.)*

having as osmolarity of 150 mosmol/L. Now, imagine that this liter of urine really consists of 500 mL of isoosmotic fluid (300 mosmol/L) and 500 mL of pure water; accordingly, the free-water clearance in this case is 500 mL, and this is the volume of pure water eliminated from the body. Another example—1 L of urine having an osmolarity of 1200 mosmol/L. Three liters of pure water would have to be *added* to this liter to make it isoosmotic; in terms of the body-fluid osmolarity, excretion of this liter of urine, therefore, has essentially the same effect as if 3 L of pure water had been added to the body, since a total of 900 mosmol of solute had been excreted above and beyond the 300 mosmol of solute required for isoosmolarity of the liter of urine. Whenever the urine is hypoosmotic, free-water clearance is said to be "positive," when it is hyperosmotic, free-water clearance is said to be "negative."[1]

To reiterate, pure-water deficits or gains are compensated by partially dissociating water excretion from that of salt through changes in ADH secretion. What receptor input controls ADH under such conditions? The answer is: changes in body-fluid osmolarity. The adaptive rationale should be obvious, since osmolarity is the variable most affected by pure-water gains or deficits. The osmoreceptors involved are located in the hypothalamus, but the mechanism by which they detect changes in osmolarity are unknown.[1] The hypothalamic cells which secrete ADH receive neural input from these osmoreceptors. Via these connections, an increase in osmolarity stimulates them and increases their rate of ADH secretion; conversely, decreased osmolarity inhibits ADH secretion (Fig. 35).

We have now described two different afferent pathways controlling the ADH-secreting hypothalamic cells, one from baroreceptors and one from osmoreceptors. These hypothalamic cells are, therefore, true integrating centers whose rate of activity is determined by the total synaptic input. Thus, a simultaneous increase in extracellular volume and decrease in extracellular osmolarity causes maximal inhibition of ADH secretion; conversely, the opposite changes produce maximal stimulation. But what happens in the following situation? A person suffering from severe diarrhea loses 3 L of salt and water during the same time that he or she drinks 2 L of pure water. The total extracellular volume is decreased, but osmolarity is also decreased. As a result, the ADH-producing cells receive opposing input from the baroreceptors and osmoreceptors. Which predominates depends completely upon the strength of the two inputs.

To add to the complexity, the ADH-secreting cells receive synaptic input from many other brain areas; thus, ADH secretion and, therefore, urine flow can be altered by pain, fear, and a variety of other factors. However, these effects are usually short-lived and should not obscure the generalization that ADH secretion is determined primarily by the states of extracellular volume and osmolarity. Alcohol is a powerful inhibitor of

[1]The formula for calculating free-water clearance is as follows:

$$C_{H_2O} = V - \frac{U_{osmol}V}{P_{osmol}}$$

where V is the urine volume per unit time, U_{osmol} is the urine osmolarity, and P_{osmol} is the plasma osmolarity. The formula was not given in the text so that the reader would be forced to deal with the concepts underlying the equation.

[1]Some evidence suggests that these receptors may actually be sodium-sensitive rather than osmoreceptors. The end result is the same, since sodium is normally the major determinant of osmolarity.

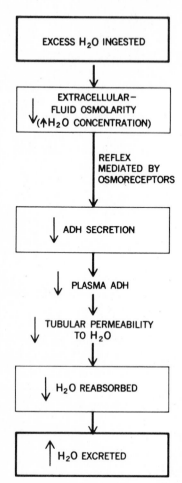

Figure 35 Pathway by which ADH secretion is lowered and water excretion raised when excess water is ingested. *(From A. J. Vander et al., Human Physiology, © 1970 by McGraw-Hill, Inc. Used with permission of McGraw-Hill Book Company.)*

ADH release—a fact that probably accounts for much of the large urine flow accompanying the ingestion of alcohol.

The disease diabetes insipidus, which is different from diabetes mellitus, or sugar diabetes, illustrates what happens when the ADH system is disrupted. Diabetes insipidus is characterized by the constant excretion of a large volume of highly dilute urine (as much as 25 L/day). In most cases, the flow can be restored to normal by the administration of ADH. These patients apparently have lost the ability to produce ADH, usually as a result of damage to the hypothalamus. Thus, distal-tubule and collecting-duct permeability to water is low and unchanging regardless of extracellular osmolarity or volume. The very thought of having to urinate (and therefore to drink) 25 L of water per day underscores the importance of ADH in the control of renal function and body-water balance.

Figure 36 shows many of the factors known to control renal sodium

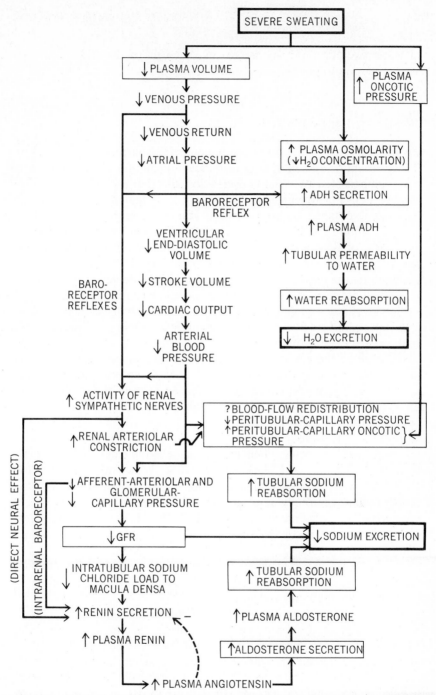

Figure 36 Pathways by which sodium and water excretion are decreased in response to severe sweating. This figure is basically an amalgamation of Figs. 26, 28–31, 34, and the converse of Fig. 35. For clarity, the possible contributions of a natriuretic hormone and the direct actions of the sympathetic nerves and angiotensin on tubular reabsorption are not shown. *(Modified from A. J. Vander et al., Human Physiology, © 1970 by McGraw-Hill, Inc. Used with permission of McGraw-Hill Book Company.)*

and water excretion in response to severe sweating, as in exercise; the renal retention of fluid helps to compensate for the water and salt lost in the sweat.

THIRST AND SALT APPETITE

Now we must turn to the other component of the balance—control of intake. It should be evident that large deficits of salt and water can be only partly compensated by renal conservation and that ingestion is the ultimate compensatory mechanism. The subjective feeling of thirst, which drives one to obtain and ingest water, is stimulated both by a reduced extracellular volume and by an increased plasma osmolarity. The adaptive significance of both are self-evident. Note that these are precisely the same changes which stimulate ADH production. The centers which mediate thirst are located in the hypothalamus and are very close to those areas which produce ADH. They are also very close to, but distinct from, food-intake centers. Damage to the thirst centers abolishes water intake completely. Conversely, electric stimulation of them may induce profound and prolonged drinking.

Because of the similarities between the stimuli for ADH secretion and for thirst, it is tempting to speculate that the receptors (osmoreceptors and atrial baroreceptors) which initiate the ADH-controlling reflexes are identical to those for thirst. This may, indeed, be the case, but there are also other pathways controlling thirst. For example, dryness of the mouth and throat causes profound thirst, which is relieved by merely moistening them. It is fascinating that when animals such as the camel (and humans, to a lesser extent) become markedly dehydrated, they will rapidly drink just enough water to replace their previous losses and then stop. What is amazing is that when they stop, the water has not yet had time to be absorbed from the gastrointestinal tract into the blood. Some kind of metering of the water intake by the gastrointestinal tract has occurred, but its nature remains a mystery.

As shown in Fig. 32, angiotensin stimulates thirst by a direct effect on the brain and constitutes one of the pathways by which thirst is stimulated when extracellular volume is decreased.

Salt appetite, which is the analogue of thirst, is also an extremely important component of sodium homeostasis in most mammals, particularly in the herbivores. It is clear that salt appetite is innate and consists of two components: hedonistic appetite and regulatory appetite. In other words, animals like salt and eat it whenever they can, regardless of whether they are salt-deficient, and, in addition, their drive to obtain salt is markedly increased in the presence of deficiency. The significance of these animal studies for humans is unclear. Salt craving does seem to occur in humans who are severely salt-depleted, but the contribution of regulatory salt appetite to everyday sodium homeostasis in normal persons is probably slight. On the other hand, humans do seem to have a strong hedonistic appetite for salt, as manifested by almost universally large intakes of sodium whenever it is cheap and readily available. Thus, the average American intake of salt is 10 to 15 g/day despite the fact that humans can survive quite normally on less than 0.5 g/day. Present evidence strongly suggests that a large salt intake may be an important contributor to the pathogenesis of hypertension.

Study questions: **28** to **42**

Chapter 8

Renal Regulation of Potassium Balance

OBJECTIVES

The student understands the renal regulation of potassium.
1 Describes the basic renal processes for handling potassium
2 Contrasts the contribution of each nephron site to potassium handling during a high- and low-potassium diet
3 Describes the mechanism by which potassium secretion is accomplished by the distal tubule
4 Lists the inputs which control the rate of potassium secretion by the distal tubule so as to regulate potassium balance homeostatically
5 Describes the pathway by which changes in potassium balance influence aldosterone secretion
6 Describes the effects of alkalosis on potassium secretion and balance
7 Describes the relationship between renal sodium handling and potassium secretion; contrasts distal-tubular secretion of potassium in persons with primary versus secondary hyperaldosteronism
8 Predicts the changes in potassium excretion and balance occurring in representative abnormal situations: respiratory or metabolic alkalosis, primary aldosteronism, diarrhea, diabetes mellitus

The potassium concentration of the extracellular fluid is a closely regulated quantity. The importance of maintaining this concentration in the internal environment stems primarily from the role of potassium in the excitability of nerve and muscle. The resting membrane potentials of these tissues are directly related to the ratio of intracellular to extracellular potassium concentration. Raising the external potassium concentration lowers the resting membrane potential, thus increasing cell excitability. Conversely, lowering the external potassium hyperpolarizes cell membranes and reduces their excitability.

Since most of the body's potassium is found within cells, primarily as a result of active-ion-transport systems located in cell membranes, even a slight alteration of rates of ion transport across cell membranes can produce a large change in the amount of extracellular potassium. Unfortunately, relatively little is known about the physiological control of these transport mechanisms except that they do play an important role in protecting against marked changes in extracellular potassium. For example, animals chronically fed a high-potassium diet manifest a greatly enhanced ability to transport potassium into cells. Both aldosterone and insulin are known to alter membrane transport of potassium in a variety of tissues, but whether they participate in either acute or chronic adaptive changes in potassium transport (such as the one just described) by nonrenal cells remains uncertain.

One important factor influencing potassium movement into many cells is the hydrogen-ion concentration of the body fluids; an increase in hydrogen-ion concentration (acidosis) is usually associated with potassium movement out of cells, and alkalosis with potassium movement into them. It is as though potassium and hydrogen ions were "exchanging" across the cell membrane (i.e., hydrogen ions moving into the cell during acidosis and out during alkalosis, with potassium doing just the opposite), but the precise mechanism underlying these "exchanges" has not yet been clarified. Moreover, these phenomena are not homeostatic mechanisms for regulating extracellular potassium but may, in fact, actually lead to profound abnormalities in potassium distribution.

Normal individuals remain in potassium balance (as they do in sodium balance) by excreting daily an amount of potassium equal to the amount of potassium ingested minus the small amounts eliminated in the feces and sweat. Normally, potassium losses via sweat and the gastrointestinal tract are small, although large quantities can be lost by the latter during vomiting or diarrhea. Again, the control of renal function is the major mechanism by which body potassium is regulated.

Potassium is completely filterable at the glomerulus.[1] The amounts of

---

[1] Recent evidence suggests that approximately 10 percent of plasma potassium may actually be protein-bound, but this is not generally accepted as yet.

potassium excreted in the urine are generally a small fraction (10 to 15 percent) of the filtered quantity. These facts establish the existence of tubular potassium reabsorption. However, it has also been demonstrated that under certain conditions the excreted quantity may actually exceed the filtered quantity. We therefore conclude that tubular potassium secretion also exists. Thus, the subject is complicated by the fact that potassium can be both reabsorbed and secreted by the tubule.

Tubular reabsorption of potassium is accomplished by active transport and occurs in the proximal tubule, ascending loop of Henle, distal tubule, and collecting duct. The quantitative contributions of the more proximal segments to reabsorption are quite similar to those for sodium. Approximately 65 percent of the total filtered potassium is reabsorbed by the proximal tubule and another 20 to 30 percent by the ascending loop of Henle.[1] Thus, only about 10 percent of the filtered potassium enters the distal tubule. Present evidence indicates that the reabsorption of this 90 percent of the filtered potassium by the proximal tubule and loop occurs at virtually the same rate regardless of changes in body potassium. In other words, the reabsorption of potassium by these nephron segments does not seem to be controlled so as to achieve potassium homeostasis.

The situation for the distal tubule and collecting ducts is quite different. First, they are able both to secrete and to reabsorb potassium.[2] Moreover, the rate at which one of these opposing processes—secretion—occurs is variable; accordingly, the *net* contribution of these nephron segments may be either reabsorption or secretion. It is by alteration of this mix in the distal tubule (and, to a lesser extent, in the collecting duct) that changes in potassium excretion are achieved.

Let us take a few examples. During potassium deprivation (caused, for example, by a low-potassium diet), the homeostatic response is to reduce potassium excretion to a minimal level. Using micropuncture to evaluate potassium handling by each nephron segment, we would find that the proximal tubule and loop were reabsorbing about 90 percent of the filtered potassium and that the distal tubule and collecting duct together were reabsorbing most of the remaining 10 percent so that very little potassium was excreted. Now we shift to the opposite end of the spec-

---

[1]Recent evidence suggests that a small amount of potassium may be *secreted* into the descending loop of Henle and, under certain conditions, into the straight portion of the proximal tubule also. Were this the case, the actual amount of potassium reabsorbed by the ascending loop of Henle would be underestimated by the figure given in the text. The entire question of the loop's handling of potassium beautifully illustrates the problems micropuncturists have in dealing with loop function and nephron heterogeneity. (See Wright and Giebisch, 1978, in Suggested Readings for Chap. 8.)

[2]Just as was the case for ADH and water permeability, it appears that the portion of distal tubule which is involved in potassium transport is the "late" portion—the "initial collecting tubule." It is not yet clear whether the "early" portion—the distal convoluted tubule—plays any role in potassium transport.

trum and look at the kidneys during a high-potassium diet. In this case the homeostatic response is to excrete large quantities of potassium so as to balance output with intake. Micropuncture reveals that the proximal tubule and the loop are still reabsorbing the same fraction (90 percent) of filtered potassium so that the amount of potassium entering the distal tubule from the loop is not much different from the amount entering it when the individual was on the low-potassium diet. Now, the radical difference appears: The distal tubule manifests net secretion of potassium rather than the net reabsorption seen on the low-potassium diet. Indeed, the quantity of potassium added to the distal lumen by secretion may be greater than the quantity of potassium reabsorbed upstream by the proximal tubule and loop. The fluid then leaves the distal tubule and flows through the collecting ducts, where a little more potassium is added by secretion. The final result is *net secretion* by the *overall nephron,* i.e., the *excretion of more potassium* than was *filtered.*

These examples should reinforce the fact that, normally, the control of renal potassium excretion resides in the distal portions of the nephron (particularly in the distal tubule), whose contribution can be either net reabsorption or secretion. It seems almost certain that the major controlled variables in these segments are those membrane transport processes which lead to secretion (see below). In other words, the membrane transport process favoring reabsorption (presumably an active potassium pump in the luminal membrane) probably operates at a relatively fixed rate despite changes in physiological conditions. A very useful simplifying assumption emerges: In describing the homeostatic control of potassium excretion, we may ignore changes in GFR or in reabsorption and focus only on the factors which alter the rate of distal potassium secretion. It must be pointed out, however, that under certain abnormal conditions, potassium reabsorption in the proximal tubule or loop may be decreased and that a large quantity of the potassium excreted may represent filtered potassium which is not reabsorbed. For example, drugs which inhibit sodium reabsorption by the proximal tubule or loop also usually inhibit potassium reabsorption at these sites (the mechanism is not clear). Another situation characterized by inhibition of proximal and loop potassium reabsorption is osmotic diuresis. Just as was true for sodium, the presence of an osmotic diuretic interferes with potassium reabsorption; this is one reason for the marked urinary loss of potassium suffered by patients with uncontrolled diabetes mellitus.

MECHANISM OF POTASSIUM SECRETION

The model for potassium secretion by the distal tubule that has been in favor for the past decade is illustrated in Fig. 37. The critical event (step 1) is the active transport of potassium from interstitial fluid across the

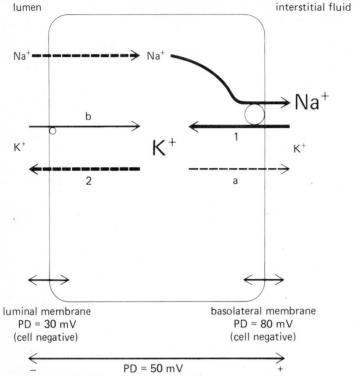

lumen   interstitial fluid

Figure 37 Diagrammatic representation of model proposed for distal tubular handling of potassium. As shown here, this cell would be secreting potassium. The dashed lines denote *net* diffusional fluxes across the individual membranes. The numbers and letters serve as guides for the text. The thicknesses of the lines are not at all drawn to scale, i.e., they serve only to emphasize which flux is greatest at each membrane, not how much greater. Note that the model is based completely on movement of potassium *through cells*, not *between* them; the tight junctions between distal-tubular cells are certainly not completely impermeable to potassium so that some small fraction of potassium secretion probably does occur across them, driven by the favorable potential difference from interstitial fluid to lumen. (This "transtubular" potential difference of 50 mV is, of course, merely the algebraic sum of the luminal and basolateral membrane potentials.)

basolateral membrane into the cell; this active transport step, which is presumed to be coupled loosely (certainly not 1:1) to active sodium extrusion via the Na-K-ATPase system, creates a very high intracellular potassium concentration so that a concentration gradient exists favoring net potassium diffusion from cell into lumen (2) [and, of course, from cell back into interstitial fluid—(a)]. Note that the concentration gradient across the luminal membrane is opposed by an electrical force (30 mV, cell-negative) which favors net diffusion from lumen to cell. However this opposing electrical force is not as large as the chemical force (the concentration gradient), and the result is net diffusion of potassium into the lumen. Thus, this model for secretion postulates active transport into the cell at the basolateral membrane and passive exit at the luminal membrane. Clearly, in such a model, activity of the basolateral pump emerges as the dominant force driving overall secretion. Note further that with the addition of a reabsorptive pump at the luminal membrane (b), one which operates at a relatively unchanging and slow rate, the cell would manifest net reabsorption rather than secretion whenever the basolateral pump activity was eliminated or greatly reduced.

Several aspects of this model remain controversial,[1] particularly the nature of the basolateral entry step. Some investigators have suggested that potassium uptake across the basolateral membrane is not by an active pump but is accounted for solely by passive diffusion driven by the 80 mV (cell-negative) potential difference generated across this membrane mainly as the result of sodium extrusion. However, several recent experiments have demonstrated that, in several conditions, free intracellular potassium concentration is too high to be achieved by the basolateral potential difference alone; accordingly, an active pump must be present.

To summarize, potassium secretion requires a cellular accumulation step at the basolateral membrane. This step is best explained by the presence of an active potassium pump, although potassium diffusion driven by the basolateral-membrane potential difference (itself dependent on active sodium transport) may also play a role. The elevated intracellular potassium concentration achieved by the basolateral accumulation step is responsible for net diffusion of potassium out of the cell into the lumen. This passive luminal step depends not only on the intracellular potassium concentration but on the luminal concentration (the other end of the concentration gradient), the magnitude of the luminal potential difference opposing diffusion into the lumen, and the permeability of the luminal membrane to potassium.

HOMEOSTATIC CONTROL OF SECRETION

What are the factors which influence distal potassium secretion so as to achieve homeostasis of body potassium? In other words, how do changes in body potassium induce the kidney to secrete more or less potassium? When a high-potassium diet is ingested (Fig. 38), plasma potassium increases, even though very slightly, and this drives enhanced basolateral uptake (either by stimulating the basolateral pump or by increasing the electrochemical gradient for passive entry). The resulting increase in intracellular potassium concentration enhances the gradient for potassium movement into the lumen and raises potassium excretion. Conversely, a

[1]See Wright, 1977, and MacKnight, 1977, in Suggested Readings for excellent reviews of all aspects of this topic.

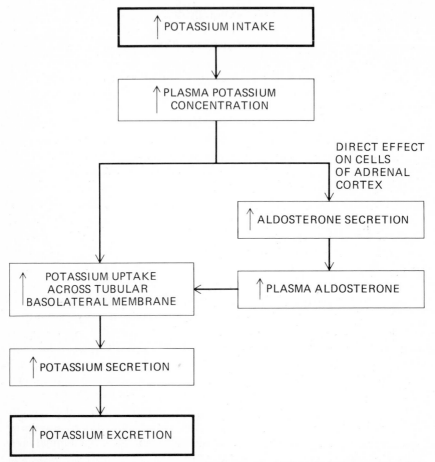

Figure 38 Pathways by which an increased potassium intake induces greater potassium excretion. The responsiveness of the renal tubules (i.e., its uptake and secretion of potassium) to increases in plasma potassium and aldosterone is significantly enhanced when the high potassium intake is chronic, an adaptation whose mechanism is not known.

low-potassium diet or a negative-potassium balance, e.g., from diarrhea, lowers renal-tubular-cell potassium concentration; this reduces potassium secretion and excretion, thereby helping to reestablish potassium balance.

A second important factor linking potassium secretion to potassium balance is the hormone aldosterone, which, besides stimulating tubular sodium reabsorption, simultaneously enhances tubular potassium secretion (Fig. 38). The reflex by which changes in extracellular volume control aldosterone production is completely different from the reflex initiated by an excess or deficit of potassium. The former constitutes a complex pathway, involving renin and angiotensin. The latter, however, seems to be much simpler and works in the following way (Fig. 39): The aldosterone-

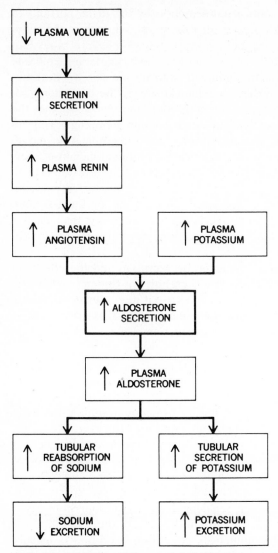

Figure 39 Summary of the control of aldosterone and its effects on renal handling of sodium and potassium. Aldosterone exerts a variety of other effects, both renal and nonrenal. Its action on tubular hydrogen-ion secretion is described in Chap. 9. *(From A. J. Vander et al., Human Physiology, © 1970 by McGraw-Hill, Inc. Used with permission of McGraw-Hill Book Company.)*

secreting cells of the adrenal cortex are apparently sensitive to the potassium concentration of the extracellular fluid bathing them (or, more likely, they are sensitive to their own intracellular potassium concentration). Thus, an increased intake of potassium leads to an increased extracellular potassium concentration, which, in turn, directly stimulates aldosterone production by the adrenal cortex. This extra aldosterone circulates to the kidney, where it increases potassium secretion by the distal portions of the nephron and, thereby, eliminates the excess potassium from the body. Aldosterone seems to influence potassium secretion in several ways, but its dominant action is probably a stimulation of the basolateral-membrane entry step (Fig. 38). (This is consistent with aldosterone's ability to stimulate sodium reabsorption, since any enhancement of the basolateral sodium pump would be expected to increase potassium entry whether the latter was directly or indirectly coupled to sodium pumping.) This increases intracellular potassium concentration and the gradient for movement into the lumen. (Aldosterone also increases luminal-membrane permeability to potassium so that the enhanced gradient for diffusion is even more effective in driving luminal entry.) Conversely, a lowered extracellular potassium concentration decreases aldosterone production and, thereby, inhibits tubular potassium secretion; less potassium than usual is excreted in the urine, thus helping to restore the normal extracellular potassium concentration.

The two major controls of aldosterone secretion and the effects of this hormone on sodium and potassium secretion are summarized in Fig. 39. It should be evident that a conflict will arise if increases in potassium and extracellular volume occur simultaneously, since these two changes drive aldosterone production in opposite directions.

OTHER FACTORS INFLUENCING POTASSIUM SECRETION

We have now described the mechanisms by which potassium secretion is controlled so as to achieve potassium homeostasis. However, the fact is that potassium secretion is also influenced by factors *not* designed to maintain body potassium constant; indeed, these factors may be so potent as to upset potassium balance. The most important of them clinically are acid-base disturbances and altered renal sodium handling[1] (particularly diuretic drugs). This is because the renal mechanisms for potassium are so intimately related to those for sodium and hydrogen ion. The empirical finding that any given factor influences potassium excretion is usually quite straightforward; in contrast, the *mechanism* by which it does so is often much less clear, but this should not be too surprising given the fact the basic mechanism of potassium secretion is still hazy. One should not lose the forest (the empirical finding) for the trees (the likely mechanisms)

---

[1]The relationship between the renal handling of sodium chloride and potassium is not a one-way street. Primary changes in potassium balance may have important effects on sodium reabsorption by multiple mechanisms. The text describes one of the indirect influences resulting from potassium-induced changes in aldosterone. There are others, including direct effects of potassium both on tubular sodium reabsorption and on renin secretion. (See Laragh and Sealey, 1973, in Suggested Readings for Chap. 7.)

in these subsequent descriptions. It is very likely that multiple mechanisms are involved in the overall action of each factor, but for simplicity only those considered most important are presented.

Acid-Base Changes

The empirical finding is as follows: The existence of an alkalosis, either metabolic or respiratory in origin, induces increased potassium secretion and excretion (Fig. 40). Thus, a primary disturbance in a person's acid-base status can result in a secondary disturbance in potassium balance. For example, a patient suffering from metabolic alkalosis (induced, say, by vomiting) will manifest increased urinary excretion of potassium solely as a result of the alkalosis and will, therefore, become potassium-deficient. Of course, as soon as potassium balance is upset by these events, the homeostatic mechanisms described in the previous section (for example, decreased aldosterone secretion) will be triggered so as to limit the imbalance.

The stimulatory effects of alkalosis on potassium secretion appear to be mediated, at least in part, through an increase in the potassium concentration of distal-tubular cells. (This same type of effect of alkalosis on nonrenal cell potassium concentration was described earlier in this chap-

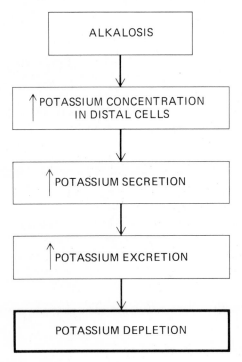

Figure 40 Pathway by which alkalosis causes potassium depletion.

ter.) It is likely that the presence of an alkalosis somehow stimulates the basolateral potassium entry step.

What about the presence of an acidosis—does it do just the opposite, i.e., reduce potassium secretion and, thereby, cause potassium retention? For respiratory acidosis and certain forms of metabolic acidosis, the answer is "yes," but only during the most acute stages (usually less than 24 h). In other forms of metabolic acidosis there may not even be an acute retention phase because some factor other than the acidosis per se is dominant. But the really surprising fact is that even respiratory acidosis and those forms of metabolic acidosis which manifest acute reductions in potassium excretion usually come ultimately to manifest *increased* potassium secretion. Attempts have been made to explain these phenomena,[1] but at the moment the fact remains that the mechanisms by which acidosis alters renal potassium handling are too poorly understood to serve as a bolster for the learning of physiological principles.

Finally, it should be emphasized that the relationships described here are only one side of the coin; we shall describe in the next chapter how primary changes in potassium balance induce secondary changes in the renal handling of hydrogen ions.

Altered Renal Sodium Handling

The empirical finding is as follows: Potassium excretion is almost always found to be increased when urinary sodium excretion is increased in the following situations: a diet very high in sodium chloride, saline infusion, osmotic diuresis, or diuretic drugs which act on the proximal tubule and/or loop of Henle (Fig. 41). The increased potassium excretion is due mainly to enhanced distal-tubular *secretion,* although as mentioned earlier in this chapter, inhibition of proximal or loop *reabsorption* may also make some contribution to increased *excretion* in all of these situations. Particularly in the last two categories, the potassium loss may be severe enough to cause serious potassium depletion.

In all these situations, the volume of fluid flowing into and through the distal tubule per unit time is increased, largely because of inhibition of sodium (or chloride) reabsorption in nephron segments proximal to the distal tubule (see Chaps. 6 and 7). It is this increase in fluid delivery to the potassium-secreting sites in the distal tubule which brings about increased potassium secretion, mainly through the following mechanism. Recall that the final step in potassium secretion—movement across the luminal membrane—is a passive process driven by the concentration gradient for potassium from cell to lumen. Because a large volume flow through the tubule (just by its diluting effect) prevents the luminal concentration from rising rapidly as potassium enters from the cell, the gra-

---

[1]See Gennari and Cohen, 1975, in Suggested Readings for Chap. 8.

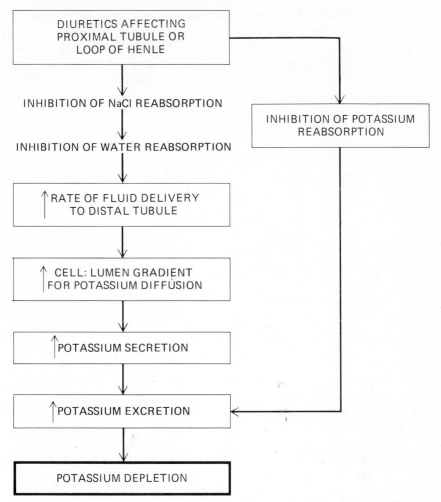

Figure 41 Pathway by which diuretic drugs affecting the proximal tubule or loop of Henle cause potassium depletion. The decrease in potassium reabsorption is a less important factor than increased secretion.

dient for passive entry is maintained at a high value, and so luminal entry is enhanced.[1]

It should be noted that in the situations listed, the increased volume flow through the distal nephron is due to increased delivery of fluid from

[1]A second possible factor linking the volume of fluid flow to potassium secretion may be the sodium in the fluid. The presence of increased amounts of sodium both in the lumen of the tubule and moving across the cells during reabsorption may enhance several of the steps in potassium secretion. For example, increased activity of the basolateral-sodium pump (secondary to the increased load of sodium) would be expected to enhance the basolateral entry step for potassium.

more proximal segments. One might have predicted that water diuresis, induced by an absence of ADH, should also cause excretion of large amounts of potassium, since it, too, causes increased fluid flow through the more distal nephron segments, but such is not the case. A major reason is that much of the effect of ADH is distal to the major flow-dependent potassium-secreting sites.

What about situations in which fluid delivery to the distal tubule is significantly *reduced* because of decreased GFR and/or enhanced sodium chloride reabsorption by the proximal tubule or loop? Because of the low volume of fluid, the secretory movement into the lumen of even relatively small amounts of potassium causes the intraluminal concentration to reach a value high enough to abolish the electrochemical gradient for further entry completely; accordingly, a decreased fluid delivery to the distal tubule tends to inhibit potassium secretion.[1] Yet despite this, in the two major types of situations which cause distal fluid delivery to be reduced—salt depletion and the diseases of secondary hyperaldosteronism with edema (see Chap. 7)—potassium secretion may be relatively unchanged rather than decreased. The reason for this is that in these situations plasma aldosterone is elevated (as described in Chap. 7), and the stimulatory effect of aldosterone on potassium secretion counterbalances the inhibitory effect of the reduced fluid delivery to the distal tubule. The net result is that such patients generally manifest relatively normal rates of potassium secretion and excretion. Contrast this to the patient with primary hyperaldosteronism; this person has an elevated aldosterone and a normal or increased delivery of fluid to the distal tubule (review the changes in renal sodium handling which occur in primary hyperaldosteronism—Chap. 7) and so suffers a marked and persistent elevation in potassium secretion and excretion, enough to cause serious potassium depletion.

Study questions: **43** to **47**

---

[1]There is at least one other reason that low flows diminish the electrochemical gradient for potassium into the lumen; sodium concentration becomes very low in such situations and this somehow causes the luminal membrane to become more polarized (cell more negative than usual relative to lumen).

Chapter 9

Renal Regulation of Extracellular Hydrogen-Ion Concentration

OBJECTIVES

The student understands the renal regulation of extracellular pH.
1 States the role of the kidneys in the regulation of extracellular pH
2 States the two ways in which the kidneys perform this role
3 Calculates the mass of bicarbonate filtered each day
4 Describes the acidifying effect of renal bicarbonate loss
5 Describes the mechanism by which tubular bicarbonate reabsorption occurs; states the role of carbonic anhydrase
6 Describes how tubular acid secretion can add new bicarbonate to the blood, i.e., lead to the excretion of hydrogen ion
7 States the limiting urine pH, the reason for it, and its significance
8 Defines titratable acid and describes how the measurement is made; states the major buffer(s) which contributes to the formation of titratable acid and its quantitative contributions
9 Describes the role of ammonia in the contribution of new bicarbonate to the blood; defines diffusion trapping and describes how it explains the relationship between urine pH and ammonium excretion; defines ammonia adaptation to chronic acidosis
10 Distinguishes the rates of acid secretion and excretion
11 Calculates, given data, the rate of total acid secretion

12 Calculates, given data, the rate at which the kidneys contribute new bicarbonate to the blood (acid excretion)

13 Describes glomerulotubular balance for bicarbonate

14 Describes the relationship between Pco_2 and tubular acid secretion

15 Lists the changes (increase or decrease) of acid secretion, titratable acid excretion, bicarbonate excretion, ammonium excretion, renal addition of new bicarbonate to the blood, and plasma bicarbonate in: metabolic acidosis, metabolic alkalosis, respiratory acidosis, respiratory alkalosis

16 Describes the influence of salt depletion on bicarbonate reabsorption and the capacity of the kidneys to repair an alkalosis

17 States the effect of increased aldosterone alone on hydrogen-ion secretion

18 States the effect of severe potassium depletion on hydrogen-ion secretion and the ability of the kidneys to compensate for a metabolic alkalosis

19 Describes how a combination of aldosterone excess and potassium depletion generates a metabolic alkalosis; given the cause of an aldosterone excess, predicts whether this excess will induce potassium depletion via the urine

20 States the effects of large amounts of cortisol or parathyroid hormone on hydrogen-ion secretion

21 Describes how primary changes in acid secretion can influence sodium and chloride reabsorption

22 Describes the urine findings in a patient treated with a carbonic anhydrase inhibitor and the mechanisms responsible

The homeostatic control of hydrogen-ion concentration in the body fluids is accomplished primarily by regulation of the carbon dioxide–bicarbonate buffer system:

$$H_2O + CO_2 \rightleftharpoons H_2CO_3 \rightleftharpoons H^+ + HCO_3^-$$

There are, of course, other buffer systems in the body, but they are all in equilibrium with each other; therefore, a change in one buffer pair causes changes in the other buffer systems. In other words, the hydrogen-ion concentration can be fixed by manipulating the concentrations of the components of a single buffer system. There are extremely precise physiological mechanisms for regulating the carbon dioxide–bicarbonate system; the Pco_2 is regulated by the respiratory system, and the bicarbonate concentration by the kidneys.

The kidneys perform their function in two major ways: (1) variable reabsorption of the bicarbonate filtered at the glomerulus, and (2) addition of *new* bicarbonate to the plasma flowing through the kidneys. As we shall see, these two processes are totally interrelated and are, in fact, accomplished by a single mechanism—tubular secretion of hydrogen ion. Inspection of the carbon dioxide–bicarbonate equation above makes it obvious how control of these two renal processes homeostatically regulates extracellular-fluid hydrogen-ion concentration. When plasma hydrogen-ion concentration has been reduced (alkalosis), it can be raised back toward normal by lowering plasma bicarbonate concentration, thereby driving the reaction to the right and generating more hydrogen ion; this the kidneys do by failing to reabsorb all the filtered bicarbonate during alkalosis, allowing this unreabsorbed bicarbonate to be excreted in the urine. *In essence, the excretion of a bicarbonate ion in the urine has virtually the same effect on the blood as would adding a hydrogen ion to the blood.* In contrast to this renal compensation for alkalosis, when plasma hydrogen-ion concentration has been increased (acidosis), the kidneys reabsorb all the filtered bicarbonate and, in addition, contribute new bicarbonate ions (produced by the renal tubular cells) to the blood, thereby shifting the reaction to the left and returning plasma pH toward normal. As we shall see, the renal addition of new bicarbonate to the blood is associated with the excretion of an equal amount of acid in the urine; "the kidney has added new bicarbonate to the blood" and "the kidney has *excreted* acid" are synonymous statements. (Throughout this section the reader must be careful to distinguish between *secretion* and *excretion*.) Thus, to compensate for acidosis, the kidneys excrete an acid urine and alkalinize the blood; in response to alkalosis, they excrete an alkaline urine and acidify the blood.

BICARBONATE REABSORPTION

Bicarbonate is completely filterable at the glomerulus. How much is normally filtered per day?

$$\text{Filtered } HCO_3^-/\text{day} = \text{GFR} \times P_{HCO_3^-}$$
$$= 180 \text{ L/day} \times 24 \text{ meq/L}$$
$$= 4320 \text{ meq/day}$$

Zero reabsorption of this bicarbonate would be tantamount to adding more than 4 L of 1 N acid to the body. In a normal person, i.e., in the absence of alkalosis, virtually all is reabsorbed. Thus, the reabsorption of bicarbonate is normally a conservation process, and essentially none appears in the urine.

How is bicarbonate reabsorbed? One might naturally assume that reabsorption of bicarbonate occurs passively as a result of the same forces described earlier for chloride, but such is the case only for a very small fraction of total bicarbonate reabsorption. There are two reasons for the relative insignificance of passive bicarbonate reabsorption: First, the combined permeability of the luminal-basolateral membranes and/or tight junctions to bicarbonate is relatively low compared to that for chloride;

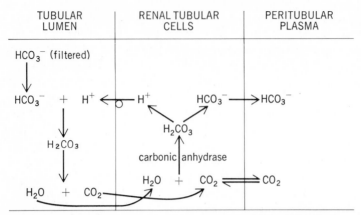

Figure 42 Mechanism by which filtered bicarbonate is reabsorbed. In studying this figure, begin with the carbon dioxide entering the cell from the peritubular plasma (for simplicity, the interstitial fluid between the basolateral membrane and peritubular capillary has been left out) and proceed upwards. In the scheme illustrated here, H^+ is generated in the cell directly by the dissociation of H_2CO_3, but the following scheme may actually be the case: The H^+ to be secreted is generated from water, and the resulting OH^- is left behind in the cell, where it reacts with CO_2 to generate HCO_3^- in a reaction catalyzed by carbonic anhydrase ($CO_2 + OH^- \xrightarrow[\text{anhydrase}]{\text{carbonic}} HCO_3^-$). The overall result—the generation of H^+ and HCO_3^- with the participation of carbonic anhydrase—is the same in either case, so we have used the one with the more familiar form of the reaction mediated by carbonic anhydrase. Also not shown in the figure is the fact that, in the proximal tubule, the breakdown of H_2CO_3 to CO_2 and H_2O in the lumen is also catalyzed by carbonic anhydrase, which is present in the luminal membrane.

second, the active-transport process for bicarbonate is so dominant that it greatly reduces any electrochemical gradient favoring net passive movement out of the lumen. (For example, it lowers luminal concentration of bicarbonate.) We will, therefore, ignore any contribution of passive bicarbonate reabsorption (i.e., passive movement all the way across the tubule from lumen to interstitium; passive movement across the basolateral membrane is, as we shall see, an integral component of the active-transport process).

The active reabsorption of bicarbonate is not accomplished in the conventional manner of simply having an active pump for bicarbonate ions.[1] Rather, the mechanism by which bicarbonate is reabsorbed involves hydrogen-ion secretion and is shown in Fig. 42. In studying this complicated figure, begin with the carbon dioxide entering the cell from the peritubular plasma and proceed upwards.

---

[1]This statement is by no means universally accepted. Some investigators have argued that as much as 40 percent of bicarbonate reabsorption is mediated by an active pump acting upon the bicarbonate ion itself (see Maren, 1974, in Suggested Readings), but the weight of evidence supports the view that such is not the case (see Malnic and Steinmetz, 1976, in Suggested Readings).

The key elements in this scheme are the intracellular hydration of carbon dioxide (catalyzed by the enzyme carbonic anhydrase) to carbonic acid, dissociation of the acid to generate hydrogen ion, and the active secretion of this hydrogen ion into the lumen. The bicarbonate generated simultaneously in the cell moves into the interstitial fluid by diffusion down its electrochemical gradient. (Recall that the cell interior is markedly negative relative to the interstitial fluid.) Once in the tubular lumen, the hydrogen ion combines with a filtered bicarbonate ion to form carbonic acid; this decomposes to water and carbon dioxide, which diffuse into the cell and then either diffuse into the peritubular plasma or are used by the cell to generate another hydrogen ion. It may seem inaccurate to refer to this process as bicarbonate reabsorption, since the bicarbonate which appears in the peritubular plasma is not the same bicarbonate ion which was filtered. Yet the overall result is, in effect, the same as it would be if the filtered bicarbonate had been more conventionally reabsorbed like a sodium or potassium ion.

It is also important to note that the hydrogen ion which was *secreted* into the lumen is *not excreted* in the urine. It has been incorporated into water and reabsorbed. The key point here is that any secreted acid (hydrogen ion) which combined with bicarbonate in the lumen to effect bicarbonate reabsorption does not contribute to the urinary *excretion* of acid.

Finally, it should be mentioned that the process of acid secretion is intimately related to sodium reabsorption. Indeed, it has been postulated that, at least in the proximal tubule, the extrusion step for hydrogen ion at the luminal membrane may be coupled to the entry of sodium (by facilitated diffusion) across this membrane. In this view, the hydrogen-ion movement is a "secondary active transport" process (see Chap. 2), using the energy from the simultaneous downhill movement of sodium in the opposite direction. At present, the weight of evidence does not favor this hypothesis, but regardless of its validity, there is absolutely no question that renal sodium handling somehow exerts profound effects on hydrogen-ion secretion, a problem to which we shall return later in this section.

The process of hydrogen-ion secretion and bicarbonate reabsorption occurs throughout the nephron with the exception of the descending loop of Henle. Quantitatively, the proximal tubule is most important in that it reabsorbs approximately 80 to 90 percent of the filtered bicarbonate. The remaining bicarbonate is normally reabsorbed by the loop of Henle and distal tubule. Throughout the tubule, as shown in Fig. 42, *intracellular* carbonic anhydrase is involved in the reactions generating hydrogen ion and bicarbonate. In the proximal tubule, carbonic anhydrase is also located in the luminal cell membranes, and this carbonic anhydrase catalyzes the *intraluminal* decomposition of the very large quantities of carbonic acid formed in this nephron segment.

ADDITION OF NEW BICARBONATE TO THE PLASMA (RENAL EXCRETION OF ACID)

Besides being able to conserve all the filtered bicarbonate, the kidneys can also contribute *new* bicarbonate to the plasma, so that the mass of bicarbonate in the renal veins exceeds that which entered the kidneys originally. The effect of adding new base to the body is, of course, to alkalinize it, and this is the renal compensation for acidosis.

The mechanism by which new bicarbonate is added to the blood is fundamentally the same as that for bicarbonate reabsorption, namely, tubular acid secretion (Fig. 43). The only difference between these two processes is a function of the fate of the secreted hydrogen ions within the tubular lumen. In the case of bicarbonate reabsorption, the secreted acid combines with filtered bicarbonate and is reabsorbed as water; whereas, in the case of new bicarbonate addition to the blood, the secreted acid combines with other buffers in the lumen (or, to an extremely small degree, remains free in solution) and is excreted. Let us first consider the case in which the secreted acid combines with phosphate, one of the two most important urinary buffers, the other being ammonia.

Note that the process of hydrogen-ion secretion is the same tubular mechanism described previously, but the net overall effect is different simply because the secreted acid reacts with filtered phosphate rather than with filtered bicarbonate. Therefore, the bicarbonate generated within the tubular cell and entering the plasma constitutes a net gain of bicarbonate by the blood, not merely a replacement for a filtered bicarbonate. Thus, when a secreted hydrogen ion combines in the lumen with a buffer other than bicarbonate, the overall effect is not merely one of

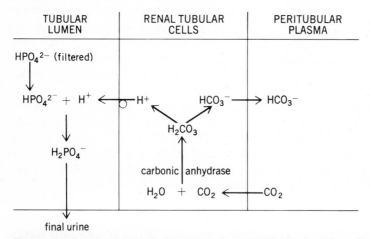

Figure 43 Reaction of secreted hydrogen ion with filtered phosphate. Note that a carbon dioxide has been used up, and a new bicarbonate has been released into the blood. In contrast, Fig. 42 shows that no net gain or loss of carbon dioxide or bicarbonate occurs when the secreted hydrogen ion is used for bicarbonate reabsorption.

bicarbonate conservation but rather of addition to the body of *new* bicarbonate, which raises the bicarbonate concentration of the blood and alkalinizes it.

The figure also demonstrates another important point; namely the renal contribution of new bicarbonate to the blood is accompanied by the *excretion* of an equivalent amount of acid in the urine. In this case, in contrast to the reabsorption of bicarbonate, the *secreted* hydrogen ion remains in the tubular fluid, trapped there by the phosphate buffer, and is *excreted* in the urine. This should reinforce the concept that, when they add new bicarbonate to the blood, the kidneys are really excreting hydrogen ion from the body, thereby alkalinizing it. The message should also be clear that the source of essentially all excreted hydrogen ion is tubular secretion. Glomerular filtration of hydrogen ions makes no significant contribution because the concentration of free hydrogen ion at a pH of 7.4, the pH of glomerular filtrate, is less than 10^{-7} M. Even multiplying this by 180 L/day, one comes up with less than 0.1 mmol filtered per day.

Figure 44 illustrates the same process but with ammonia rather than phosphate as the intraluminal buffer. Unlike phosphate, ammonia gains entry to the tubular lumen not by filtration but rather by tubular synthesis and secretion, the mechanism of which will be described later. Again we see that the overall effect is the addition of new bicarbonate to the plasma, combination of the secreted acid with an intraluminal buffer, in this case ammonia, and excretion of the acid.

The type and quantity of buffers is a crucial determinant of the maximal rate at which the kidneys can contribute new bicarbonate to the blood. This stems from the fact that net addition of hydrogen ions to the lumen ceases when a maximal luminal hydrogen-ion concentration is reached. The reasons for this differ in the proximal and distal tubules. The former, as we have seen, has a relatively leaky epithelium, and, therefore,

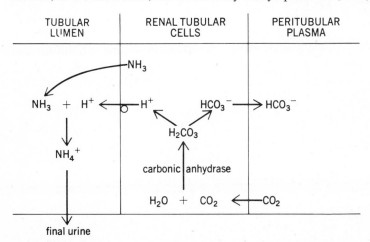

Figure 44 Reaction of secreted hydrogen ion with ammonia formed by tubular cells.

manifests "pump-leak" characteristics; as the luminal hydrogen-ion concentration rises due to the active entry of hydrogen ions, the gradient for passive diffusion of hydrogen ions from lumen to interstitial fluid increases. Accordingly, a point is reached at which the passive efflux from the lumen exactly equals the active influx from the cells, and no further net addition can occur. In contrast, the distal tubule is much less "leaky," and so diffusion out of the lumen is not really a problem. Rather, the existence of a maximal concentration in this nephron segment is accounted for by the fact that the active luminal pump itself is directly inhibited in the presence of a low pH; it virtually ceases to operate when the pH reaches 4.4. This value is considerably lower than the minimal pH achievable by the proximal tubule and, therefore, sets the minimal pH achievable in the final urine. Accordingly, the nature and quantity of urinary buffers available to react with the secreted acid and prevent this limiting concentration for free hydrogen ion from being reached is of key importance.

Phosphate as a Buffer

The relationship between monobasic and dibasic phosphate is as follows:

$$HPO_4^{2-} + H^+ \rightleftharpoons H_2PO_4^-$$

This buffer pair provides an excellent buffer system because its pK is 6.8. Expressed in Henderson-Hasselbach terms:

$$pH = 6.8 + \log \frac{[HPO_4^{2-}]}{[H_2PO_4^-]}$$

At the normal pH of plasma and, therefore, of the glomerular filtrate, the equation becomes

$$7.4 = 6.8 + \log \frac{[HPO_4^{2-}]}{[H_2PO_4^-]}$$

Solving the equation, we find that there is four times more dibasic (HPO_4^{2-}) than monobasic ($H_2PO_4^-$) phosphate in plasma. Therefore, the HPO_4^{2-} is available for buffering secreted hydrogen ions. By the time the minimal pH of 4.4 is reached, virtually all the HPO_4^{2-} has been converted to $H_2PO_4^-$.

How much HPO_4^{2-} is normally filtered per day?

$$\begin{aligned}
\text{Filtered total phosphate/day} &= 180 \text{ L/day} \times 1 \text{ mmol/L}[1] \\
&= 180 \text{ mmol/day} \\
\text{Filtered } HPO_4^{2-} &= 80\% \times 180 \text{ mmol/day} \\
&= 144 \text{ mmol/day}
\end{aligned}$$

[1]This number, 1 mM, is the value of phosphate in glomerular filtrate; it is somewhat lower than the plasma concentration because a small fraction of plasma phosphate is protein-bound and, therefore, not filterable.

However, not all of this filtered HPO_4^{2-} is available for buffering, because about 75 percent of filtered phosphate is reabsorbed. Accordingly, unreabsorbed HPO_4^{2-} available for buffering is 0.25×144 mmol/day = 36 mmol/day. Thus, the reabsorption of phosphate considerably limits the supply of HPO_4^{2-} for buffering.[1] Accordingly, as we shall see, ammonia must usually bear the major burden of accepting the additional hydrogen ions in acidosis.

Ammonia and phosphate are normally the only important urinary buffers. However, under abnormal conditions, certain organic buffers may appear in the tubular fluid in large enough quantity to allow them also to act as important buffers. A particularly interesting example is the patient with uncontrolled diabetes mellitus. As a result of insulin deficiency, such a patient may become extremely acidotic because he produces large quantities of acetoacetic and β-hydroxybutyric acid, which, at plasma pH, almost completely dissociate to yield anions (β-hydroxybutyrate and acetoacetate) and hydrogen ions. These anions are filtered at the glomerulus but are only partly reabsorbed because they are present in great enough quantities to exceed the renal reabsorptive T_m's for them. Accordingly, they are available in the tubular fluid to buffer a portion of the acid being secreted by the tubules to compensate for the acidosis. However, their usefulness in this role is limited by the fact that their pK's are low—approximately 4.5. This means that only half of these anions will be titrated by secreted acid before the limiting urine pH of 4.4 is reached; i.e., only half of them can actually be used as buffers. If the kidneys could lower the luminal pH to 1, as the stomach can, then it could titrate all of the β-hydroxybutyrate.

Ammonia as a Buffer

The ammonia-ammonium reaction has a very high pK, approximately 9.2:

$$NH_3 + H^+ \rightleftharpoons NH_4^+$$
$$pH = 9.2 + \log \frac{[NH_3]}{[NH_4^+]}$$

This means that, given the usual urine pH of 7.4 or less, virtually all NH_3 that gains entry to the tubular lumen will immediately pick up hydrogen ions to form NH_4^+. Accordingly, as long as a supply of NH_3 is available, hydrogen-ion secretion and net addition of bicarbonate to the blood can continue with no danger of reaching the minimal urinary pH.

Ammonia Synthesis and Diffusion Trapping

The glomerular filtrate is not a significant source of ammonia because its combined concentration of NH_3-NH_4^+ is very low, and only about 1 per-

[1]Logically, it would seem that a good homeostatic response would be to have phosphate reabsorption inhibited by the presence of acidosis so that more luminal phosphate would be available for buffering; however, this does not actually occur.

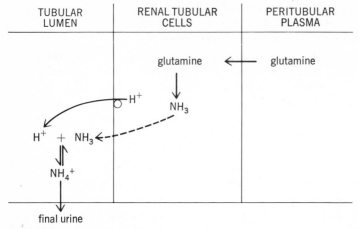

| TUBULAR LUMEN | RENAL TUBULAR CELLS | PERITUBULAR PLASMA |

Figure 45 Ammonia synthesis and entry into the tubular lumen. (See text for pathways leading to synthesis of ammonia.)

cent of even this small amount is in the form of NH_3. (The plasma pH is 7.4 and the reaction pK is 9.2.) Accordingly, the source of ammonia is the renal tubular cells themselves, glutamine serving as the major precursor[1] (Fig. 45). The deamidation and deamination of glutamine and its metabolites to yield ammonia proceeds by a variety of metabolic pathways, some in the cytosol and others in the mitochondria, but the single most important one seems to be that mediated by mitochondrial glutaminase.[2]

When an individual is acidotic for more than a few days, there occurs a marked increase in ammonia synthesis. This phenomenon, known as *adaptation of ammonia synthesis,* involves enhanced transport of glutamine into mitochondria and/or increased activity of glutaminase. (These changes are probably not mediated by a direct effect of the acidosis on the renal tubules but rather by an as yet unidentified chemical messenger, the release of which is stimulated by the acidosis.) The result of this adaptation is that the increased ammonia synthesis provides more ammonia to act as intraluminal buffer, so the kidneys can compensate for the chronic acidosis by contributing a larger amount of new bicarbonate to the blood.

The mechanism by which ammonia, once having been synthesized within the cell, gains entry to the lumen is of considerable importance (Fig. 45). It is known as *nonionic diffusion,* or *diffusion trapping,* and its

[1]Considering the importance of plasma glutamine in ammonia synthesis, it is surprising that we know little concerning its site of origin (presumably mostly skeletal muscle) or the control of its synthesis during acid-base disorders.

[2]In this pathway, the conversion of a molecule of glutamine to α-ketoglutarate generates two hydrogen ions as well as ammonia. Therefore, for ammonia production to actually facilitate net elimination of hydrogen ions from the body, these two hydrogen ions must be eliminated by metabolism of the α-ketoglutarate to glucose (recall that renal tubular cells are capable of gluconeogenesis) or by its complete oxidation to CO_2 and water.

underlying principles were previously described in Chap. 3 in the context of tubular handling of organic solutes. Recall that the ability of a substance to penetrate any cell membrane passively depends upon the lipid solubility of the substance. Accordingly, ammonia, being nonionized, is highly lipid-soluble; whereas ammonium, being charged, is highly lipid-insoluble. Thus, ammonia readily diffuses across the renal-cell membranes, whereas ammonium does not. The synthesis of ammonia within the cell creates a cell-lumen concentration gradient down which ammonia diffuses. (Obviously, ammonia will diffuse into the blood also, but we ignore this for the sake of simplicity.) In both the cell and lumen, there exists an equilibrium between ammonia and ammonium. The key point is that the relative amounts of each member of this buffer pair present in the cell and lumen depend upon pH. When the tubular fluid is acid, what happens to the ammonia after it diffuses into the lumen? Immediately, almost all of the ammonia combines with hydrogen ion to form ammonium. Thus, the ammonium concentration in the lumen increases, but since the membrane is virtually impermeable to ammonium, it is trapped within the lumen. Since the ammonia is converted to ammonium almost as fast as it enters, the concentration of ammonia in the lumen is kept low, and the concentration gradient from cell to lumen is maintained. (This assumes that ammonia synthesis keeps pace with exit so as to maintain the intracellular concentration.)

Thus, ammonia passively diffuses into the lumen and is trapped there by conversion to ammonium. The lower the pH of the tubular fluid, the more effective this process, and the more ammonia that enters the lumen. It should be clear, therefore, that this process forces an efficient coupling between renal tubular acid secretion and the supply of buffer (ammonia) required to react with the secreted hydrogen ion. As the pH of the tubular fluid decreases because of increased acid secretion, the falling pH automatically induces increased entry and trapping of ammonia in the lumen with subsequent buffering of the hydrogen ions. As long as ammonia synthesis by the cells can keep up with demand (i.e., unbuffered hydrogen ions in the lumen), then hydrogen-ion secretion can continue without causing the tubular pH to reach the minimal limiting value. The fact that increased ammonia synthesis occurs during chronic acidosis (the adaptation process described above) permits ammonia to serve as the major urinary buffer in the kidneys' compensation for acidosis. Ammonium excretion may increase from a normal value of 20 meq/day to 500 meq/day in a person suffering from severe acidosis. In contrast, phosphate's contribution may increase by only 20 to 40 meq/day.

The other side of this coin should also be emphasized: When the urine is not acid, there will be very little diffusion trapping of ammonia. Unless enough acid is secreted by the tubules to force a significant reduction of tubular-fluid pH, little ammonium will be excreted in the urine.

QUALITATIVE INTEGRATION OF BICARBONATE
REABSORPTION AND ACID EXCRETION

To reiterate, acid secreted by the tubules can suffer one of two general fates: (1) It can combine with filtered bicarbonate, in which case the overall process accomplishes bicarbonate reabsorption. (2) Or it can combine with filtered nonbicarbonate buffers such as phosphate or with ammonia that has been synthesized and secreted by the tubules.

The first case is a conservation process, by which the kidneys prevent loss of bicarbonate from the body. This process alone does not alkalinize the body but rather prevents the development of an acidosis due to bicarbonate loss. In contrast, the second process contributes new bicarbonate to the body and simultaneously excretes acid, thereby alkalinizing it.

What determines whether the secreted hydrogen ions, once in the lumen, combine with bicarbonate, on the one hand, or with phosphate, ammonia, or organic buffers, on the other? This depends upon the pK's of each buffer-pair reaction and upon the mass of each buffer present. To simplify matters, one may assume that, compared to bicarbonate, relatively little nonbicarbonate buffer is titrated, i.e., combines with hydrogen ion, until most of the bicarbonate has been reabsorbed. This phenomenon occurs largely because the quantity of bicarbonate is huge compared to the quantity of the other buffers. Once most of the filtered bicarbonate has been reabsorbed, then almost all of the secreted acid combines with the other buffers.

One can imagine, then, a spectrum of events reflecting the acid-base status of the body.

Alkalosis

When an alkalosis exists, the kidneys compensate by secreting too little acid to accomplish complete reabsorption of filtered bicarbonate. Therefore, bicarbonate is excreted in an alkaline urine, and the body is thereby made more acid. Simultaneously, because the acid secreted is inadequate to reabsorb all the bicarbonate, there is virtually no hydrogen ion available to combine with nonbicarbonate buffers. This is just what one would expect teleologically, since the kidneys are "attempting" to eliminate bicarbonate from the body, not add new bicarbonate to it.

Normal State

Metabolism of the average American diet results in the net liberation of 40 to 80 meq of hydrogen ion per day. Therefore, if balance is to be maintained, the kidneys must excrete this same amount of acid, i.e., contribute 40 to 80 meq of new bicarbonate to the blood. (Again, we emphasize that these are synonymous statements.) Accordingly, tubular acid secretion must be great enough to effect complete reabsorption of all filtered bicarbonate, and an additional 40 to 80 meq acid must be secreted to contribute 40 to 80 meq new bicarbonate to the blood, this acid being excreted in the urine buffered by phosphate and ammonia. The urine under such circumstances is moderately acid, perhaps at pH 6.

Acidosis

The kidneys compensate for acidosis by adding large quantities of new bicarbonate to the blood. Therefore, as in the previously described normal state, acid secretion must be great enough to effect complete reabsorption of all filtered bicarbonate. Beyond this, the tubules must secrete large amounts of additional acid so as to add an equivalent amount of new bicarbonate to the blood. This acid is excreted in the urine buffered by phosphate and ammonia and by organic buffers, when they are present. Under such conditions, ammonia usually becomes the most important buffer; its supply by diffusion trapping is assured by the fact that once all the bicarbonate is reabsorbed, the large continued secretion of acid causes the tubular-fluid pH to fall progressively.

These generalizations should also make it easy to visualize the general pattern of pH changes as fluid flows through the proximal and distal tubules. Most of the hydrogen ions secreted into the proximal-tubular lumen go for reabsorption of bicarbonate (simply because so much bicarbonate is filtered), only a small amount of nonbicarbonate buffers are titrated, and the drop in luminal pH is relatively small, usually no more than 1 pH unit. In contrast, as fluid flows through the distal tubule, the small amount of bicarbonate remaining is soon reabsorbed, and most of the secreted hydrogen ions combine with nonbicarbonate buffers. As titration of these buffers reaches completion, the luminal pH decreases to values much lower than those which existed in the proximal tubule. It is, therefore, highly adaptive that, as we have seen, the distal tubule has a much lower limiting pH than does the proximal.

It should now be clear how, via changes in the rate of a single variable, namely, the rate of tubular acid secretion, the kidneys can compensate for the entire range of acid-base patterns which can occur. The factors which regulate this process in response to acid-base changes will be discussed after the following section detailing the methods for *quantitating* renal handling of hydrogen ion.

QUANTITATION OF RENAL ACID-BASE FUNCTIONS
Measurement of Tubular Acid-Secretion Rate

A hydrogen ion secreted by the tubules can combine in the lumen with bicarbonate, phosphate, ammonia, or one of several organic buffers. In order to calculate the total mass of acid secreted per unit time, one must add up the contributions of all these pathways. The amount of free hydrogen ion may be ignored because it is so small.

It is worthwhile to emphasize once more the great difference between the fate of a hydrogen ion reacting with bicarbonate and the fate of one reacting with any of the other buffers. As described above, the combination of a hydrogen ion with bicarbonate causes the generation of carbon dioxide and water, both of which are reabsorbed by the tubules. Thus, the secreted hydrogen ion that is used for bicarbonate reabsorption does not remain in the urine. How, then, can one measure it? The answer reflects the fact that one bicarbonate ion is reabsorbed as a result of the secretion of one hydrogen ion. Therefore, assuming this one-to-one ratio, we can calculate the mass of secreted hydrogen ion reacting with bicarbonate by measuring the rate of bicarbonate reabsorption. The rate is equal to the difference between filtered and excreted bicarbonate. For example, given the following data, how much secreted acid combined in the lumen with bicarbonate?

$$\left. \begin{array}{l} \text{GFR} = 180 \text{ L/day} \\ P_{HCO_3^-} = 24 \text{ meq/L} \\ \text{Urine vol} = 1 \text{ L/day} \\ U_{HCO_3^-} = 24 \text{ meq/L} \end{array} \right\} \text{Basic data}$$

$$\begin{aligned} \text{Filtered } HCO_3^-/\text{day} &= \text{GFR} \times P_{HCO_3^-} \\ &= 180 \text{ L/day} \times 24 \text{ meq/L} \\ &= 4320 \text{ meq/day} \\ \text{Excreted } HCO_3^-/\text{day} &= U_{HCO_3^-} \times V \\ &= 24 \text{ meq/L} \times 1 \text{ L/day} \\ &= 24 \text{ meq/day} \\ \text{Reabsorbed } HCO_3^-/\text{day} &= \text{filtered } HCO_3^-/\text{day} - \text{excreted } HCO_3^-/\text{day} \\ &= 4320 \text{ meq/day} - 24 \text{ meq/day} \\ &= 4296 \text{ meq/day} \end{aligned}$$

Thus, 4296 meq H^+ must have been secreted to accomplish the reabsorption of 4296 meq HCO_3^-.

In contrast to the hydrogen ion which reacts with bicarbonate, that which combines with phosphate or organic buffers does remain in the tubular fluid and is excreted in the urine bound to the buffers. This quantity of acid can be measured by taking a sample of urine and titrating it with sodium hydroxide back to pH of 7.4, the pH of the plasma from which the glomerular filtrate originated. This simply reverses the events which occurred within the tubular lumen when the tubular fluid was titrated by secreted hydrogen ions. Thus, the number of milliequivalents of sodium hydroxide required to reach pH 7.40 must equal the number of milliequivalents of hydrogen ion added to the tubular fluid which combined with phosphate and the organic buffers. This value is known as the *titratable acid*.

It must be stressed that the titratable-acid measurement does *not* pick up hydrogen ions which combined with ammonia to yield ammonium. The reason is that the pK of the ammonia-ammonium reaction is so high (9.2) that titration with alkali to pH 7.4 will not remove the hydrogen ions from the ammonium. In addition to measuring titratable acid, therefore, a separate measurement of urinary ammonium excretion must be performed.

The total rate of tubular hydrogen-ion secretion is thus equal to the sum of:

HCO_3^- reabsorption meq/time
+titratable acid, meq/time
+NH_4^+ excretion, meq/time

Values for a person on a normal diet are approximately:

HCO_3^- reabsorption = 4300 meq/day
Titratable acid = 20 meq/day
NH_4^+ excretion = 40 meq/day

These values serve to emphasize that the vast majority of secreted hydrogen ions are used to accomplish bicarbonate reabsorption, with only a small number remaining for the production of titratable acid or ammonium.

Measurement of Renal Contribution of New Bicarbonate to the Blood

The above analysis also indicates how to calculate the amount of *new* bicarbonate added to the blood by the kidneys, an extremely important number, since it is a precise measurement of the degree to which the kidneys have alkalinized the body. It is simply the sum of titratable acid and ammonium. (Again, the amount of free hydrogen ion may be ignored because it is so small.) This sum measures the rate of acid *excreted* in the urine secondary to tubular acid secretion, and, as we have stressed several times, it is identical to the quantity of new bicarbonate added by the renal tubular cells to the blood. This stems from the fact that each hydrogen ion secreted into the lumen which reacts with a nonbicarbonate buffer remains in the tubular fluid and is excreted.

We can now state the data required for a quantitative assessment of the renal contribution to acid-base regulation in any patient:

---

1 Titratable acid excreted

2 + NH_4^+ excreted

3 − HCO_3^- excreted (i.e., filtered HCO_3^- lost from the body because of incomplete reabsorption)

Total = net HCO_3^- gain or loss to the body (negative values equal loss, positive values equal gain).

Typical urine data for the renal compensations in the three states described are as follows:

Alkalosis

$$
\begin{array}{rl}
\text{Titratable acid} = & 0 \text{ meq/day} \\
+ \ NH_4^+ = & 0 \text{ meq/day} \\
- \ HCO_3^- \text{ excreted} = & \underline{-80 \text{ meq/day}} \\
& 80 \text{ meq } HCO_3^- \text{ } lost \text{ from the body} \\
& (\text{Urine pH} = 8.0)
\end{array}
$$

Normal state

$$
\begin{array}{rl}
\text{Titratable acid} = & 20 \text{ meq/day} \\
+ \ NH_4^+ = & 40 \text{ meq/day} \\
- \ HCO_3^- \text{ excreted} = & \underline{-1 \text{ meq/day}} \\
& 59 \text{ meq } HCO_3^- \text{ } added \text{ to the body} \\
& (\text{Urine pH} = 6.0)
\end{array}
$$

Acidosis

$$
\begin{array}{rl}
\text{Titratable acid} = & 40 \text{ meq/day} \\
+ \ NH_4^+ = & 160 \text{ meq/day} \\
- \ HCO_3^- \text{ excreted} = & \underline{0 \text{ meq/day}} \\
& 200 \text{ meq } HCO_3^- \text{ } added \text{ to the body} \\
& (\text{Urine pH} = 4.6)
\end{array}
$$

Note, however, that data shown for alkalosis are typical for respiratory alkalosis and for "pure" metabolic alkalosis, i.e., alkalosis uncomplicated by other electrolyte abnormalities. As we shall see in subsequent sections, other electrolyte imbalances frequently complicate the picture in metabolic alkalosis so that the urine may not be alkaline.

HOMEOSTATIC CONTROL OF RENAL TUBULAR ACID SECRETION

There are multiple factors which control the key element in the kidney's acid-base machinery, the rate of tubular acid secretion. Several of these factors control acid secretion so as to homeostatically regulate the pH of the body fluids.

Glomerulotubular Balance for Bicarbonate

One of the important influences on hydrogen secretion is analogous to the phenomenon of glomerulotubular balance previously described for sodium. Hydrogen secretion (and, therefore, bicarbonate reabsorption) varies directly with GFR. For example, if GFR increases 25 percent, so does bicarbonate reabsorption. The adaptive value of such a relationship is that changes in GFR do not induce potentially serious perturbations in the acid-base status of the body. In the example of the 25 percent increase cited above, if acid secretion and bicarbonate reabsorption did not increase proportionally to GFR, a very large quantity of bicarbonate would be lost from the body with a resulting acidosis. The mechanism responsible for bicarbonate glomerulotubular balance is not clear at present but very likely is part of the same overall process which achieves glomerulotubular balance for sodium.

Pco₂ and Renal Intracellular pH

The most important single determinant of the rate of tubular acid secretion, so far as homeostatic regulation is concerned, is the Pco_2 of the arterial blood. As shown in Fig. 46, the rate of hydrogen-ion secretion, as manifested by bicarbonate reabsorptive rate, is directly related to the Pco_2 of the arterial plasma. (In this figure, bicarbonate reabsorption is expressed in milliequivalents per 100 mL GFR rather than in milliequivalents per time because of the previously described influence of glomerulotubular balance.) This relationship holds over the entire range of arterial Pco_2 values.

There are no nerves or hormones mediating this response; rather, the renal tubular cells respond to the Pco_2 of the blood perfusing them. An increased Pco_2 of arterial blood causes, by diffusion of carbon dioxide, an

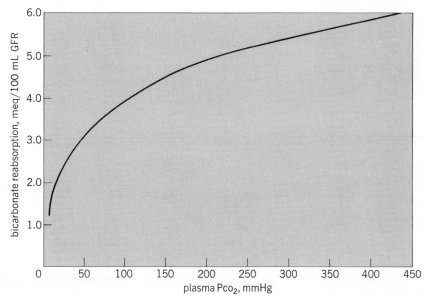

Figure 46   The relationship between Pco_2 of arterial blood and reabsorption of bicarbonate in the dog. [*Data from F. C. Rector, Jr., et al., J. Clin. Invest.,* **39**:*1706 (1960).*]

equivalent increase in P_{CO_2} within the tubular cells. This causes an increased rate of formation of carbonic acid and, in turn, an elevated intracellular hydrogen-ion concentration. Presumably, it is this change that directly stimulates the rate of hydrogen-ion secretion. In other words, the ultimate stimulus for hydrogen-ion secretion is not the P_{CO_2} per se but rather the decreased intracellular pH it induces.

The reason that intracellular pH is so responsive to changes in arterial P_{CO_2} is the ease with which carbon dioxide diffuses across cell membranes. Thus, a small change in blood P_{CO_2} causes an almost immediate equivalent change in cell P_{CO_2}, which, by mass action, alters cell pH.[1] In contrast to this sensitivity to P_{CO_2} changes, cell pH is much less dependent upon changes in blood pH per se—the reasons being that cell membranes are less permeable to the diffusion of hydrogen ion itself (or of bicarbonate) and that transport mechanisms for hydrogen ion at the basolateral membrane can minimize the transmission of extracellular pH changes into the cell. This is not to say that the cells are completely impervious to extracellular pH changes unaccompanied by simultaneous changes in P_{CO_2}. Such extracellular pH changes (particularly when chronic) generally do influence intracellular pH but much less than extracellular P_{CO_2} changes do. Accordingly, the rate of renal acid secretion correlates better with blood P_{CO_2} than with blood pH.

Renal Compensation for Respiratory Acidosis and Alkalosis

Let us apply this analysis to the clinical situations, respiratory acidosis and alkalosis. For reference, we shall present the basic equations again. (CO_2 rather than H_2CO_3 can be used in the second equation because their concentrations are always in direct proportion to one another.)

$$H_2O + CO_2 \rightleftharpoons H_2CO_3 \rightleftharpoons H^+ + HCO_3^-$$

$$[H^+] = K \frac{[CO_2]}{[HCO_3^-]}$$

In chronic pulmonary insufficiency, carbon dioxide is retained, and the resulting increase in P_{CO_2} drives the carbon dioxide–bicarbonate reaction to the right, with a resulting acidosis. It should be clear from both equations that the pH could be restored to normal if the bicarbonate could be elevated to the same degree as the P_{CO_2}. There is, of course, an automatic increase in bicarbonate concentration solely as a result of the reaction being driven to the right, but this is not nearly to the same degree

---

[1]This effect of P_{CO_2} on intracellular pH is not the only way in which P_{CO_2} influences acid secretion. Recent evidence suggests that some of its influence is not exerted directly on the kidney at all but is the indirect consequence of altered cardiovascular function. (See Arruda and Kurtzman, 1978, in Suggested Readings.)

as the rise in P_{CO_2}. If we transpose the second equation, we can see why mass action does not lead to proportionate increases of bicarbonate and carbon dioxide:

$$[H^+] [HCO_3^-] \rightleftharpoons K[CO_2]$$

This form of the equation emphasizes that a rise in carbon dioxide causes a proportionate rise in the *product* $[H^+]$ $[HCO_3^-]$. Since hydrogen-ion concentration increases, bicarbonate concentration cannot increase as much as carbon dioxide does or else their product would rise more than proportionally. (Plug in some numbers and convince yourself this is true.)

It is the kidneys' job to cause the additional bicarbonate increase by contributing new bicarbonate to the blood. This occurs because the increased P_{CO_2} stimulates renal tubular acid secretion so that all filtered bicarbonate is reabsorbed and much secreted acid is left over for the formation of titratable acid and ammonium, i.e., for the addition of new bicarbonate to the blood. This process continues until a new steady state is reached, at which point the plasma bicarbonate is now so high that even the enhanced rate of acid secretion can serve only to reabsorb the increased filtered load of bicarbonate and cannot contribute large amounts of new bicarbonate. The renal compensation is not usually perfect; i.e., when the steady state is reached, the plasma bicarbonate is not elevated to quite the same degree as is the P_{CO_2}. Consequently, blood pH is not completely returned to normal.

The sequence of events in response to respiratory alkalosis is just the opposite. As a result of hyperventilation, the patient transiently eliminates carbon dioxide faster than it is produced, thereby lowering his P_{CO_2} and raising pH. The decreased P_{CO_2} reduces tubular acid secretion so that bicarbonate reabsorption is not complete. Bicarbonate is then lost from the body, and the loss results in a decreased plasma bicarbonate and a return toward normal pH.

Renal Compensation for Metabolic Acidosis and Alkalosis

The primary cause of so-called metabolic acidosis is either the addition to the body (by ingestion, infusion, or production) of increased amounts of acid other than carbonic acid or, alternatively, the loss from the body of bicarbonate (as in diarrhea). Inspection of the equations reveals that either loss of bicarbonate or addition of hydrogen ions will lower both the plasma pH and the plasma bicarbonate concentration. The kidney compensation is to raise the plasma bicarbonate concentration back toward normal, thereby returning pH toward normal. In order to do this, the kidneys must reabsorb all the filtered bicarbonate and contribute new bicarbonate through the formation of titratable acid and ammonium. This is precisely what normal kidneys do, and the urines excreted in respiratory and metabolic acidosis are indistinguishable in these respects.

Yet the surprising fact is that in metabolic acidosis (in contrast to respiratory acidosis), these events occur in the absence of a significant stimulus to the kidney to increase acid secretion; indeed, they frequently occur in the presence of a decreased stimulus, since the P_{CO_2} of arterial blood, which is the major stimulus for tubular acid secretion, as described above, is *not increased* in metabolic acidosis but is usually *decreased*. Why? Because, as the arterial pH falls as a result of whatever is causing the metabolic acidosis, pulmonary ventilation is reflexly stimulated. This is, of course, the respiratory compensation for the acidosis, and its effect is to reduce arterial P_{CO_2}. Therefore, because renal-tubular-cell pH is rapidly altered by changes in P_{CO_2}, renal-tubular-cell pH is likely to be *increased* in the early stages of metabolic acidosis. (In patients with chronic metabolic acidosis, it is likely that intracellular pH returns to normal or actually decreases, despite a continued decrease in P_{CO_2}, probably because of altered basolateral-membrane transport of hydrogen ion.)

How, then, can the kidneys manage to perform their compensatory function with no stimulus to increase acid secretion? This apparent paradox is resolved when one recalls that in uncompensated metabolic acidosis the plasma bicarbonate is lower than normal. (In contrast, during respiratory acidosis plasma bicarbonate is greater than normal, even in the uncompensated state.) Therefore, the mass of bicarbonate filtered is reduced proportionally to the decreased plasma bicarbonate, and less hydrogen ion need be secreted to accomplish its total reabsorption. Accordingly, even with a decreased total acid secretion, there is still considerable hydrogen ion available after the bicarbonate has been completely reabsorbed to form large amounts of titratable acid and ammonium, i.e., to contribute new bicarbonate to the plasma. For example, compare the data for a person with metabolic acidosis with those for a normal person:

		Normal	*Metabolic acidosis*
Plasma HCO_3^-	Basic data	24 meq/L	12 meq/L
GFR		180 L/day	180 L/day
Filtered HCO_3^-		4320 meq/day	2160 meq/day
1 Reabsorbed HCO_3^-		4315 meq/day	2160 meq/day
2 Titratable acid and NH_4^+		60 meq/day	200 meq/day
3 Total H^+ secreted [(1) + (2)]		4375 meq/day	2360 meq/day

Thus, even in the presence of a greatly reduced acid secretion, the kidneys are able to compensate for the metabolic acidosis. Indeed, the limiting factor in this type of acidosis turns out to be not the rate of acid secretion but rather the availability of buffer. For example, in the situation of metabolic acidosis just described, although their ability to secrete hydrogen ion may well have been somewhat reduced by the presence of a low P_{CO_2}, the tubules could certainly have secreted more than 2360 meq if more buffer were available.

The situation in metabolic alkalosis is just the opposite; despite a normal or increased rate of acid secretion (secondary to a reflexly elevated P_{CO_2}) the load of filtered bicarbonate is so great that much bicarbonate escapes reabsorption,[1] and no titratable acid or ammonium can be formed. Therefore, plasma bicarbonate is decreased, and pH decreases toward normal.

OTHER FACTORS INFLUENCING HYDROGEN-ION SECRETION

The previous section described the mechanisms by which hydrogen-ion secretion is controlled so as to achieve acid-base homeostasis. We now describe how factors not designed to maintain pH constant can also influence hydrogen-ion secretion and bicarbonate reabsorption. In other words, just as was true for potassium, hydrogen-ion balance has its own distinct homeostatic controls, but it is also at the mercy of other interacting factors. The most important of these are aldosterone, extracellular-volume contraction, and potassium depletion. (Again, similarly to potassium, such interactions are the result of the close interlinking of renal sodium, potassium, chloride, and hydrogen-ion handling.) These factors may have two general effects: First, they may cause the kidneys to generate an acid-base disorder in the body by secreting too much or too little hydrogen ion; second, their presence may not cause the kidneys to generate an acid-base disorder but may prevent them from doing their usual job of compensating for an already existing acid-base disorder.

Influence of Salt Depletion on Acid Secretion

The presence of salt depletion and extracellular-volume contraction interferes with the ability of the kidneys to compensate for a metabolic alkalosis. In metabolic alkalosis, the plasma bicarbonate is elevated, either because of addition of bicarbonate to the body or because of loss of acid from it. The normal renal compensation should be to set hydrogen-ion secretion at a level which fails to achieve complete bicarbonate reabsorption and thereby allows the excess bicarbonate to be excreted. But the presence of the salt depletion not only stimulates sodium reabsorption but also stimulates hydrogen-ion secretion. The actual mechanisms by which

---

[1]Recent experiments suggest that during metabolic alkalosis, not only does some bicarbonate escape reabsorption, but there may actually occur *secretion* of bicarbonate ions into the collecting ducts. If this proves to be true, the overall picture of renal bicarbonate handling will obviously require reevaluation.

the salt depletion enhances hydrogen-ion secretion are unclear at present, but the effect is mainly on proximal hydrogen-ion secretion.[1] The net result is that all of the filtered bicarbonate is reabsorbed so that the already elevated plasma bicarbonate associated with the preexisting metabolic alkalosis is locked in, and the plasma pH remains unchanged; instead of being alkaline as it should, the urine is somewhat acid.

It should be emphasized that salt depletion will not usually induce the kidneys to generate a metabolic alkalosis; rather, it merely reduces their ability to compensate for a metabolic alkalosis once the alkalosis is established from some other cause. The major reason that salt depletion alone does not *cause* an alkalosis is that it usually has relatively little stimulating effect on the distal tubule's generation of titratable acid and ammonium. In other words, sodium depletion induces complete reabsorption of filtered bicarbonate but little or no renal contribution of new bicarbonate. If the plasma bicarbonate level is normal to start with, reabsorption of all the filtered bicarbonate along with sodium merely maintains the same normal plasma bicarbonate level. It does not increase plasma bicarbonate level. The situation is analogous to the reabsorption of glucose in normal individuals; i.e., reabsorption of all the filtered glucose merely keeps plasma glucose at the normal level.

Finally, it should be noted that we have referred to salt depletion in this section without distinguishing between sodium and chloride losses. This is because loss of either of these ions will lead to extracellular-volume contraction. (There has been considerable controversy concerning a possible specific additional effect of chloride deficiency, but no clear-cut answer is available.)

Aldosterone and Potassium Depletion

This section offers an excellent example of how two distinct inputs, each relatively small by itself, can together produce a major effect of great clinical significance. First we will consider the individual effects.

Aldosterone (as well as other mineralocorticoids), when present at a high blood concentration, stimulates hydrogen-ion secretion by a direct action on the distal tubules and collecting ducts.[2] This effect seems to be quite distinct from aldosterone's actions on sodium reabsorption and potassium secretion even though the same nephron segments are involved. By itself, this effect is quite small and has little, if any, significant effect on acid-base balance.

Potassium depletion, by itself, also tends to stimulate tubular

---

[1]A distal-tubular effect can also be revealed with appropriate experimental manipulations but does not make an important contribution in most clinical situations associated with salt depletion.

[2]Both aldosterone and potassium depletion stimulate ammonia synthesis, but whether these constitute an important component of their effects on hydrogen-ion secretion and excretion remains unclear. (See Tannen, 1977, in Suggested Readings.)

hydrogen-ion secretion. Presumably, potassium depletion of renal tubular cells causes a decrease in renal-cell pH (because of the reciprocal relations between cell pH and potassium described in the previous chapter), and it is this which stimulates hydrogen-ion secretion. For many years, it has been argued whether potassium depletion, by itself, can stimulate tubular hydrogen-ion secretion enough to seriously alter the renal contribution to acid-base balance. Most evidence now indicates that this is the case, but only when the degree of potassium depletion is extremely severe. Such depletion can impair the kidneys' ability to repair a metabolic alkalosis because it prevents the compensatory excretion of bicarbonate.

Now we come to the critical point. The combination of potassium depletion of even moderate degree and high levels of aldosterone acts synergistically to markedly stimulate tubular hydrogen-ion secretion. As a result, the renal tubules not only reabsorb all filtered bicarbonate but contribute inappropriately large amounts of new bicarbonate to the body, thereby causing the development of metabolic alkalosis. Note that there may have been nothing wrong with the acid-base balance to start with: The alkalosis is actually generated by the kidneys themselves. (Of course, if alkalosis were already present due to some other cause, the presence of this high-aldosterone–potassium-depletion combination would not only prevent the kidneys from compensating but would make the alkalosis worse.)

This phenomenon is important because the combination of a markedly elevated aldosterone and potassium depletion occurs in a variety of clinical situations. One reason for their coexistence is that the former often causes the latter! Recall from Chap. 8 that aldosterone stimulates potassium secretion; therefore, a very high level of aldosterone may cause potassium depletion via the urine. The potassium depletion and high aldosterone then act together to induce the kidneys to generate an alkalosis. A good example of this is the patient with primary hypersecretion of aldosterone due to an adrenal tumor (Fig. 47).

However, it is essential to recognize that not all patients with high levels of aldosterone will develop potassium depletion as a consequence. This point was developed in Chap. 8 and is worth repeating here. Recall that the major stimulus for aldosterone secretion is increased activity of the renin-angiotensin system; further, that the major causes of increased renin secretion are sodium depletion and the diseases of secondary hyperaldosteronism (such as congestive heart failure), characterized by edema formation and continuous stimulation of sodium-retaining reflexes. In all these situations, even very large amounts of aldosterone fail to cause increased urinary potassium loss because there is a low flow of fluid into and through the distal segments of the nephron; this low flow reduces potassium secretion and offsets the stimulatory effects of aldosterone.

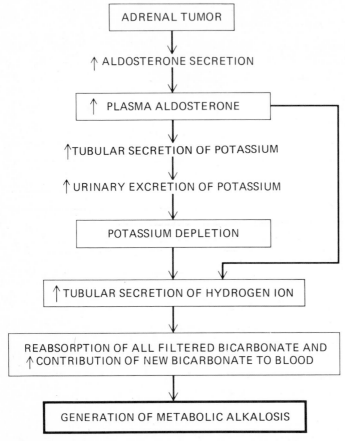

Figure 47 Pathway for generation of metabolic alkalosis in a patient with primary hyperaldosteronism. The increased aldosterone is itself the cause of the potassium depletion.

Emphasizing this point could lead to a misconception—that people with salt depletion or secondary hyperaldosteronism never have a coexisting potassium depletion. This is quite false. All we have said is that in these situations, the elevated aldosterone will not itself cause the potassium depletion, but it is quite common for something other than the aldosterone to cause potassium depletion in these patients. For example, overzealous use of diuretic drugs (Fig. 48) brings about both salt depletion (leading to increased aldosterone) and potassium depletion (as described in Chap. 8). This combination can then act to generate a metabolic alkalosis. Note also that the person in this example is doubly in trouble—as described in the previous section of this chapter, salt depletion per se (via mechanisms unrelated to aldosterone) stimulates reabsorption of bicarbonate and, therefore, helps to maintain the alkalosis once the high-aldosterone–potassium-depletion combination has generated it.

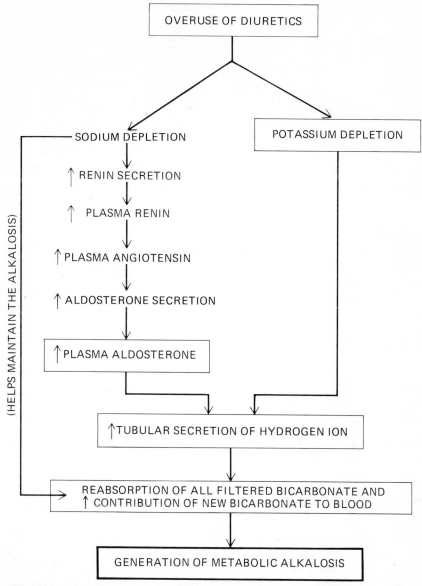

Figure 48 Pathway by which overuse of diuretics leads to a metabolic alkalosis. In contrast to the previous figures, the elevated aldosterone is not the cause of the potassium depletion. Note also that the salt depletion, via a nonaldosterone mechanism, helps to maintain the alkalosis once it has been generated.

Given the ability of aldosterone excess and potassium depletion to generate metabolic alkalosis, one might logically predict that the combination of pathologic aldosterone deficiency and potassium retention (the latter usually due to the former) might induce metabolic acidosis by partially inhibiting renal tubular secretion of hydrogen ion. Such is, in fact, the case, as illustrated by the modest metabolic acidosis manifested by patients with the inability to secrete aldosterone normally.

Cortisol and Parathyroid Hormone

A number of hormones other than aldosterone are capable of influencing tubular hydrogen-ion secretion when they are present in very high concentrations. Of these, the most important clinically are cortisol and parathyroid hormone. Cortisol's actions are quite similar to those of aldosterone and probably simply reflect the fact that high concentrations of this hormone, physiologically a glucocorticoid, can exert mineralocorticoid effects: sodium retention, potassium depletion, and metabolic alkalosis.

Parathyroid hormone's major physiological role as regulator of calcium homeostasis will be described in the next chapter. For some time it has been clear that, quite distinct from its actions on calcium, parathyroid hormone can inhibit hydrogen-ion secretion by the proximal tubule, resulting in excessive loss of bicarbonate via the urine and the development of a metabolic acidosis. This may be an important influence in patients who have excessive blood concentrations of parathyroid hormone, and some investigators believe that the response occurs at low enough concentrations for it to be a normal physiological regulator of acid-base balance; this latter hypothesis remains to be proven.

INFLUENCE OF HYDROGEN-ION SECRETION ON SODIUM CHLORIDE REABSORPTION

The previous sections described how alterations in salt balance could influence hydrogen-ion secretion. This section deals with the reverse phenomenon, the ability of primary changes in hydrogen-ion secretion and bicarbonate reabsorption to alter sodium and chloride handling.

As mentioned earlier, some investigators believe hydrogen-ion secretion (at least in the proximal tubule) to be directly coupled to the countertransport of sodium, i.e., that sodium is literally exchanged for hydrogen ion across the luminal membrane. This view makes it easy to visualize that, were hydrogen-ion secretion inhibited, sodium reabsorption would also decrease. However, even if no such *direct* coupling exists, sodium reabsorption is, in part, *indirectly* coupled by electrical forces to hydrogen-ion secretion. This indirect electrical coupling stems from the fact that bicarbonate ions constitute approximately 25 percent of the anions in the glomerular filtrate. Unless bicarbonate ions were reabsorbed at close to the same rate as sodium, there would occur a large separation of charge and a marked increase in the negativity of the tubular lumen—an event which would strongly retard further net sodium reabsorption. In

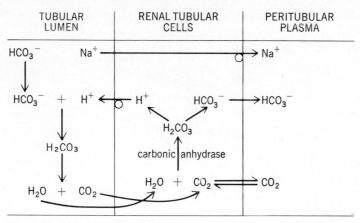

Figure 49 Tubular sodium-hydrogen exchange during reabsorption of bicarbonate.

fact, as we have seen, bicarbonate reabsorption normally occurs at the same rate as, or faster than, sodium reabsorption; since the bicarbonate is reabsorbed as a result of hydrogen-ion secretion, there is, in a sense, the "exchange" of a secreted hydrogen ion for a reabsorbed sodium ion (Fig. 49).[1]

This type of exchange occurs not only when the secreted hydrogen ion achieves bicarbonate reabsorption but also when the hydrogen ion is used in the formation of titratable acid and ammonium. Note (Fig. 50) that in both cases the titration of HPO_4^{2-} to $H_2PO_4^-$ or of NH_3 to NH_4^+ produces a net gain of one positive charge in the lumen, thereby permitting a sodium ion to be reabsorbed simultaneously with no change in intraluminal charge.

In effect, then, sodium is reabsorbed either with chloride or in exchange for hydrogen ion. There are several very important implications of these relationships for sodium chloride reabsorption:

1 There is usually an inverse correlation between the excretion rates of chloride and bicarbonate. Most simply viewed, when sodium reabsorption is proceeding relatively more rapidly than acid secretion and bicarbonate reabsorption, then more chloride will accompany the reabsorbed sodium (because of increased luminal negativity). Therefore, less chloride will be excreted. Conversely, when the rate of acid secretion is high enough so that filtrated bicarbonate is totally reabsorbed and large quantities of titratable acid and ammonium are formed, then less chloride is reabsorbed, since a larger fraction of the sodium is reabsorbed in exchange for hydrogen ion. Increased renal excretion of chloride is, there-

[1]There are reasons other than electrical coupling by which hydrogen-ion secretion and bicarbonate reabsorption influence sodium reabsorption; see Suggested Readings for Chap. 4.

CONTROL OF RENAL TUBULAR ACID SECRETION

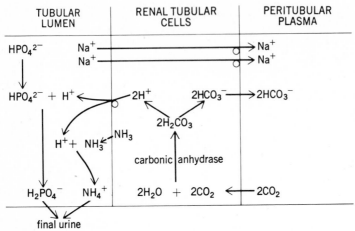

Figure 50 Tubular sodium-hydrogen ion exchange during formation of titratable acid and ammonium.

fore, one of the reasons that plasma chloride tends to go down during the renal compensation for a metabolic acidosis.

2   Whenever tubular acid secretion is inadequate to effect complete bicarbonate reabsorption, there is usually the obligatory excretion of some sodium in the urine along with the bicarbonate. However, the loss of sodium is usually not as great as the loss of bicarbonate because alkalosis also induces increased potassium secretion, as described above, and the secretion of potassium ions into the lumen allows an equivalent amount of sodium to be reabsorbed with no change in intraluminal potential. An interesting example of this phenomenon is the renal response to administration of drugs which inhibit renal carbonic anhydrase. Inhibition of this enzyme reduces acid secretion, which in turn reduces bicarbonate reabsorption. The net result is an increased excretion of sodium, bicarbonate, and water. (Unreabsorbed solute always causes the excretion of increased amounts of water.) In addition, the inhibition of carbonic anhydrase alkalinizes the renal tubular cells. (The reason for this can be deduced from the legend for Fig. 42.) The increased intracellular pH induces an enhanced secretion of potassium so that a large fraction of the excreted bicarbonate is accompanied by potassium rather than by sodium.

Study questions: **48** to **53**

Chapter 10

Regulation of Calcium Balance and Extracellular Concentration

OBJECTIVES

The student understands the regulation of calcium balance and extracellular concentration.

1   States the normal plasma calcium concentration and the percent which is protein-bound; states the effect of pH on the free fraction
2   Lists the effector sites for calcium homeostasis and the effects of parathyroid hormone, vitamin D, and calcitonin on them
3   Describes the control of secretion of parathyroid hormone and calcitonin
4   Describes the sequence of reactions leading from 7-dehydrocholesterol to $1,25\text{-}(OH)_2D_3$; states two major controls over the 1-hydroxylation step
5   Describes the effects of parathyroid hormone and vitamin D on phosphate and the ways in which they contribute to regulation of plasma phosphate concentration
6   Describes the direct and indirect effects of an increased plasma calcium concentration on renal calcium handling; describes how changes in sodium influence renal calcium handling
7   Predicts changes in plasma and urinary calcium and phosphate in patients with hyperparathyroidism or with vitamin D deficiency
8   States the effects of cortisol and growth hormone on calcium balance

Extracellular calcium concentration is normally maintained within very narrow limits, the requirement for precise regulation stemming primarily from the profound effects of calcium on neuromuscular excitability. A low calcium concentration increases the excitability of nerve and muscle cell membranes so that patients with diseases in which low calcium occurs suffer from *hypocalcemic tetany,* characterized by skeletal muscle spasms, which can be severe enough to cause death by asphyxia. Hypercalcemia is also dangerous because it causes cardiac arrhythmias as well as depressed neuromuscular excitability.

It is important to recognize that the plasma calcium (normally 5 meq/L or 2.5 mmol/L) is approximately 40 percent protein-bound. Since only the free, i.e., ionized, calcium exerts effect on nerve, muscle, and other target organs, any factor which influences the degree of protein binding can increase or decrease the effects of calcium. One of the most important influences on binding is the plasma pH. An increase in pH causes increased calcium binding because the decreased acidity converts more of the protein to the anionic form; i.e., it exposes additional negatively charged binding sites. Thus, a patient with alkalosis is extremely susceptible to tetany; whereas a patient with acidosis will not manifest tetany at levels of total plasma calcium low enough to cause symptoms in normal people.

EFFECTOR SITES FOR CALCIUM HOMEOSTASIS

Our earlier chapters on ion and water homeostasis were concerned almost entirely with the renal handling of these substances. It was possible to do so for several reasons: (1) Although internal exchanges (between extracellular fluid, on the one hand, and bone and cells, on the other) are important for these substances, the major homeostatic controls act via the kidneys. (2) Absorption of these substances from the gut approximates 100 percent under normal circumstances and is not a major controlled variable. Neither of these statements holds true for calcium homeostasis. Accordingly, this section must deal not only with the renal handling of calcium but with the other two major effector sites for calcium homeostasis—bone and the gastrointestinal tract.

Gastrointestinal Tract

The gastrointestinal tract indiscriminately absorbs virtually the total quantity of many ingested substances. But this is not true for calcium absorption, whose active-transport system is subject to quite precise hormonal control. Normally, the *net* absorption of calcium amounts to only 10 percent of that ingested, the remainder being excreted in the feces. However, the situation is complex, since the intestinal epithelium secretes considerable amounts of endogenous calcium into the lumen.

$$\begin{aligned}
\text{Ca ingested} &= 1000 \text{ mg/day} \\
\text{Ca secreted into intestinal lumen} &= \underline{600 \text{ mg/day}} \\
\text{Total in intestinal lumen} &= 1600 \text{ mg/day} \\
\text{Absorbed from gut} &= \underline{700 \text{ mg/day}} \\
\text{Excreted in feces} &= 900 \text{ mg/day}
\end{aligned}$$

In this example, 100 mg of new calcium is added to the blood each day, i.e., 10 percent of the ingested calcium. Note, however, that if gut absorption were reduced to 600 mg/day, then none of the ingested calcium would have been retained. Conversely, retention could potentially be increased tenfold were absorption raised to 1600 mg/day. Finally, lowering the rate of absorption to 500 mg/day would result in the fecal loss of 1100 mg/day; i.e., the person would go into negative calcium balance. As we shall see, control of gut calcium absorption constitutes a very important homeostatic mechanism for regulating total body balance and extracellular concentration.

Kidney

The kidneys handle calcium by filtration and reabsorption. Only about 60 percent of the plasma calcium is filterable, the remainder being protein-bound. The reabsorption process is active, occurs throughout the nephron (with the likely exception of the descending loop of Henle), and normally approximates 99 percent. The 1 percent which escapes reabsorption amounts to approximately 100 mg/day, a quantity equal to the normal net addition of new calcium to the body via the gastrointestinal tract. Thus, just as was true for the other ions discussed in this book, the kidneys help maintain a constant balance of total body calcium by matching output to intake; when intake is altered, the rate of excretion is homeostatically altered. However, it must be acknowledged that the generalizations expressed in the preceding sentence come close to exaggeration, for the kidney responds to changes in dietary calcium much less than to changes in sodium, water, or potassium. For example, it has been estimated that only about 5 percent of an increment in dietary calcium appears in the urine; at the other end of the spectrum, when dietary intake of calcium is reduced to extremely low levels, there is a slow reduction of urinary calcium, but some continues to appear in the urine for weeks.

How do the renal homeostatic mechanisms, modest as they may be, operate? Since calcium is filtered and reabsorbed, but not secreted:

$$\text{Ca excretion} = \text{Ca filtered} - \text{Ca reabsorbed}$$

Accordingly, excretion can be altered homeostatically by changing either the filtered load or the rate of reabsorption. Both occur. For example, what happens when a person increases his calcium intake? Transiently, intake exceeds output, positive calcium balance ensues, and plasma calcium concentration increases. This in itself increases the filtered mass of calcium and increases excretion. Simultaneously, as we shall see, the increased plasma calcium triggers hormonal changes which cause a diminished reabsorption. The net result of these responses is increased calcium excretion.

A bewildering array of factors not designed to maintain calcium homeostasis can also influence urinary calcium excretion, mainly by stimulating or inhibiting tubular reabsorption. These include a large number of hormones, ions, acid-base disturbances, and drugs (see Suggested Readings). Without question, the most important of them is sodium. Under most circumstances, the fractional reabsorptive rates of sodium and calcium parallel each other, and large changes in calcium excretion can be induced simply by administering or withholding salt. (This fact is made use of clinically when one wishes to increase or decrease the amount of calcium in the body.) Indeed, changes in dietary sodium are far more effective in altering urinary calcium excretion than are changes in dietary calcium. Clearly, there must be some kind of coupling between sodium reabsorption and calcium reabsorption, at least in the proximal tubule and loop of Henle. In contrast, these two ions can be dissociated in the more distal nephron segments, since their major hormonal controls—aldosterone (sodium) and parathyroid hormone (calcium)—stimulate distal reabsorption only of one ion without affecting the other.

Bone

The activities of the gastrointestinal tract and the kidneys determine the net intake and output of calcium for the entire body and, thereby, the overall state of calcium balance. In contrast, interchanges of calcium between extracellular fluid and bone do not alter total body balance but, rather, the distribution of calcium within the body. Approximately 99 percent of the total body calcium is contained in bone, which is basically a collagen-protein framework upon which calcium phosphate (and other minerals) are deposited in a crystal structure known as *hydroxyapatite*. Bone is not at all a dead, fixed tissue; rather, it is quite cellular and well supplied with blood. Most important, it is continuously broken down (resorbed) and simultaneously reformed under the influence of the bone cells. Thus, bone provides a huge potential source or sink for the withdrawal or deposit of calcium from extracellular fluid. We shall see that several hormones exert important effects on the deposition or resorption of bone calcium.

HORMONAL CONTROL OF EFFECTOR SITES

Parathyroid Hormone

All three of the effector sites described above are subject to direct or indirect control by a polypeptide hormone called parathyroid hormone, produced by the parathyroid glands. Parathyroid-hormone production is controlled directly by the calcium concentration of the extracellular fluid bathing the cells of these glands. Lower calcium concentration stimulates parathyroid-hormone production and release, and a higher concentration does just the opposite. It should be emphasized that extracellular calcium concentration acts directly upon the parathyroids without any intermediary hormones or nerves. (Recall that this is also true of the relation between extracellular potassium and aldosterone production.)

Parathyroid hormone exerts at least four distinct effects on calcium homeostasis (Fig. 51):

1   It increases the movement of calcium (and phosphate) from bone into extracellular fluid by stimulating bone resorption. In this manner the immense store of calcium contained in bone is made available for the regulation of extracellular calcium concentration.

2   It stimulates the activation of vitamin D (see below), and this latter hormone then increases intestinal absorption of calcium (and phosphate). Thus, the long-known ability of parathyroid hormone to stimulate intestinal absorption of these ions is not due to a direct action of it on the gut but rather is indirect and mediated by vitamin D.

3   It increases the renal tubular calcium reabsorption (by an action on the distal nephron) and thus decreases urinary calcium excretion.

4   It reduces the renal tubular reabsorption of phosphate, thereby raising urinary phosphate excretion and lowering extracellular phosphate concentration. (Maximal amounts of parathyroid hormone can change the percent of filtered phosphate reabsorbed from 80 to 15 percent.)

The adaptive value of the first three effects should be obvious: They all result in a higher extracellular calcium concentration and thus compensate for the lower concentration, which originally stimulated parathyroid-hormone production. The adaptive value of the fourth effect can be understood in terms of phosphate homeostasis. When parathyroid hormone induces bone reabsorption, both calcium and phosphate are released; similarly, its intestinal effect (via vitamin D) is to enhance the absorption of both calcium and phosphate. Accordingly, while the low calcium, which triggered the increase in parathyroid hormone, is being homeostatically compensated, the plasma phosphate would be raised above normal; the latter does not occur because of parathyroid hormone's inhibition of tubular phosphate reabsorption. Indeed, so potent is this ef-

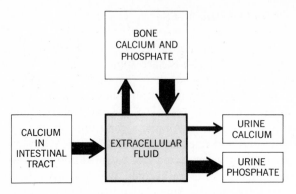

INCREASED PARATHYROID HORMONE

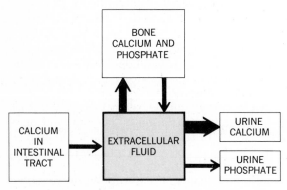

DECREASED PARATHYROID HORMONE

Figure 51 Effects of physiological changes in parathyroid hormone on the gastrointestinal tract, kidneys, and bone; the arrows signify relative magnitudes. The effect of parathyroid hormone on the intestine is not direct but is mediated by vitamin D, the action of which is controlled by the parathyroid hormone. Note that when parathyroid hormone is decreased, there is net movement of calcium and phosphate into bone, urine calcium is raised, and gastrointestinal absorption of calcium is reduced. *(From A. J. Vander et al., Human Physiology, © 1970 by McGraw-Hill, Inc. Used with permission of McGraw-Hill Book Company.)*

fect that plasma phosphate is usually reduced when parathyroid-hormone levels are elevated. (This reduction in phosphate is adaptive in that it facilitates further bone resorption because of local interactions between calcium and phosphate.)

In contrast to the state described above, an increase in extracellular calcium concentration inhibits normal parathyroid-hormone production and, thereby, produces increased urinary and fecal calcium loss and net movement of calcium from extracellular fluid into bone (Fig. 51).

Parathyroid hormone has other functions in the body, but the four effects discussed above constitute the major mechanisms by which it integrates various organs and tissues in the regulation of extracellular calcium concentration. Another candidate to join these four was described in Chap. 9—parathyroid hormone's inhibition of proximal-tubular hydrogen-ion secretion and, thereby, bicarbonate reabsorption.[1] The result of this effect is an increased extracellular-fluid hydrogen-ion concentration (acidosis), which is known to displace calcium from plasma protein (as described above) and from bone; thus, free plasma calcium concentration rises. Whether this effect of parathyroid hormone is really important at physiological plasma levels of the hormone is still not settled.

Hyperparathyroidism, due to a primary defect in the parathyroid glands (e.g., a hormone-secreting tumor), well illustrates the actions of parathyroid hormone. The excess hormone causes enhanced bone resorption, leading to bone thinning with the formation of completely calcium-free areas or cysts. Plasma calcium increases and plasma phosphate decreases; the latter is caused by increased phosphate excretion. The increased plasma calcium is deposited in various body tissues, including the kidneys, where stones are formed. A seeming paradox is that calcium excretion is increased. (Contrast this to the decreased calcium excretion induced by *physiological* amounts of parathyroid hormone— Fig. 51.) This occurs despite the fact that tubular calcium reabsorption is enhanced by parathyroid hormone. The explanation is that because of the elevated plasma calcium induced by parathyroid hormone, the filtered load of calcium increases even more than does reabsorptive rate— another excellent illustration of the necessity of taking both filtration and reabsorption into account when analyzing excretory changes.

Vitamin D

Vitamin D plays an important role in calcium metabolism, as attested by the fact that its deficiency results in poorly calcified bones. The term vitamin D denotes a group of closely related sterols. One of these compounds, now called vitamin D_3, is formed by the action of ultraviolet radiation on 7-dehydrocholesterol in the skin. Vitamin D_3, however, is inactive and must undergo metabolic changes before it can influence its target cells. It enters the blood and is hydroxylated in the 25 position by the liver and then in the 1 position by the kidneys. The end result is the active form of vitamin D—1,25-dihydroxy vitamin D_3, abbreviated $1,25\text{-}(OH)_2D_3$. From this description, it should be evident that the vitamin D formed in this way is actually a hormone, not a vitamin, since it is made in the body. Humans, because of clothing and decreased out-of-doors life, are often dependent upon dietary vitamin D for some of their supply, but this di-

[1]Parathyroid hormone also inhibits reabsorption of other solutes by the proximal tubule, including sodium and, surprisingly, even calcium. Its facilitation of distal reabsorption of calcium is, however, more potent so that the overall effect on the entire tubule is to enhance calcium reabsorption.

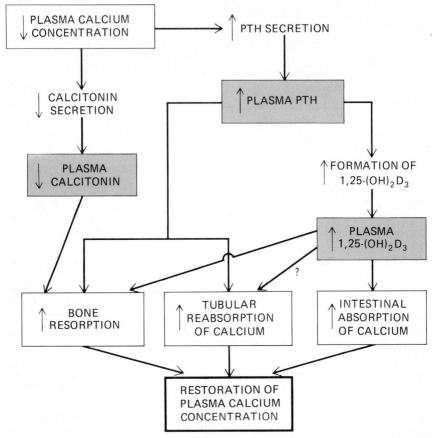

Figure 52 Hormonally mediated compensatory response to reduced plasma calcium concentration. PTH = parathyroid hormone. Urinary loss of calcium is reduced not only by the hormonally mediated increase in reabsorption shown in the figure but also because glomerular filtration of calcium is diminished due to the decrease in plasma calcium concentration.

etary vitamin D must undergo the same hepatic and renal activation as does the vitamin D_3 produced in the skin.

The major action of vitamin D is to stimulate active absorption of calcium (and phosphate) by the intestine. Thus, the major event in vitamin D deficiency is decreased gut calcium absorption, resulting in decreased plasma calcium. In children, the newly formed bone protein matrix fails to be calcified normally because of the low plasma calcium, leading to the disease *rickets*.

In addition to its effect on intestinal calcium absorption, vitamin D also significantly enhances bone resorption. The mechanism underlying this effect is unclear but may involve a facilitation by vitamin D on the bone-resorption effect exerted by parathyroid hormone. Finally, vitamin

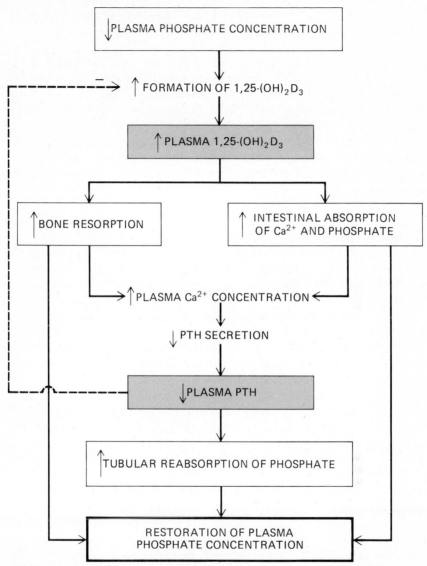

Figure 53 Hormonally mediated compensatory response to reduced plasma phosphate concentration. PTH = parathyroid hormone. Note that the decrease in PTH secretion induced by the increased plasma calcium exerts a negative-feedback "damping" effect on 1, 25-$(OH)_2D_3$ formation (signified by the dashed line ———→), that is, opposed to the stimulatory effect of the decreased phosphate. Urinary phosphate loss is decreased not only by the hormonally mediated increased reabsorption shown in the figure but also because glomerular filtration of phosphate is diminished due to the decrease in plasma phosphate concentration. Also not shown in the figure is the fact that tubular reabsorption of phosphate may also be increased directly by 1,25-$(OH)_2D_3$.

D can also stimulate the renal tubular reabsorption of calcium (and phosphate), but whether this effect is significant physiologically remains unsettled.

The blood concentration of the active form of vitamin D—1,25-$(OH)_2D_3$—is subject to physiological control. The major control point is the final hydroxylation step, which occurs in the kidneys. This step is stimulated by parathyroid hormone, a phenomenon which is highly adaptive, for it provides a mechanism for simultaneously altering the levels of these mediators in the same direction. Thus, a low plasma calcium concentration stimulates the secretion of parathyroid hormone, which, in turn, enhances the activation of vitamin D, and both substances contribute to the restoration of the plasma calcium to normal (Fig. 52).

Parathyroid hormone is not the only modulator of 1,25-$(OH)_2D_3$ formation. Phosphate is another important one.[1] In this case, an increased plasma phosphate *inhibits* formation; conversely, decreased phosphate stimulates it. This is obviously adaptive in terms of phosphate homeostasis—decreased phosphate increases activation of vitamin D, which then enhances both phosphate absorption from the gut and release from bone (and, possibly, its reabsorption by the renal tubules), with a resulting compensatory increase in plasma phosphate (Fig. 53).

Finally, the recognition that the kidneys perform the key hydroxylation step in the activation of vitamin D has clarified why patients with renal disease generally manifest a serious deficiency of vitamin D, even when they are given large amounts of precursors of 1,25-$(OH)_2D_3$. The damaged kidneys are simply unable to perform the activation step normally, and the result is a marked decrease in intestinal absorption of calcium. In contrast, therapy with 1,25-$(OH)_2D_3$ results in dramatic improvement.

Calcitonin

Yet a third hormone, calcitonin, has significant effects on plasma calcium. Calcitonin is secreted by cells within the thyroid gland which surround, but are completely distinct from, the thyroxine-secreting follicles. The calcitonin-secreting cells are called, therefore, *parafollicular cells*. Calcitonin lowers plasma calcium primarily by inhibiting bone resorption. Its secretion is controlled directly by the calcium concentration of the plasma supplying the thyroid gland; an increased calcium causes increased calcitonin secretion. Thus, this system constitutes another feedback control over plasma calcium concentration (Fig. 52). However, its overall contribution to calcium homeostasis is minor compared to that of parathyroid hormone.

---

[1]Many other possible inputs are presently being studied. For example, it is likely that estrogen and prolactin also stimulate formation of 1,25-$(OH)_2D_3$; this would be adaptive in assuring increasing gut absorption of calcium and phosphate during pregnancy.

Other Hormones

Parathyroid hormone, calcitonin, and vitamin D are the only hormones whose production rates are known to be altered as part of homeostatic responses to calcium balance. However, several other hormones do influence calcium, so that changes in their rates of secretion can produce calcium imbalances. Thus, high levels of cortisol can induce negative calcium balance by depressing gut absorption of calcium while increasing its renal excretion. Growth hormone also increases urinary calcium excretion, but it simultaneously increases gut absorption. The net effect of these counterbalancing influences of growth hormone is usually a positive calcium balance.

Study questions: **54** and **55**

Study Questions

1 The difference between outer-cortical (superficial) and inner-cortical (juxtamedullary) nephrons is that the former have their glomeruli in the cortex whereas the glomeruli of the latter arise in the medulla. True or false?

False. All glomeruli are in the cortex. See text for description.

2 When a patient is given a drug which inhibits "converting enzyme," there is little physiological effect because the decrement in angiotensin II (and III) is compensated for by the simultaneous rise in angiotensin I. True or false?

False. Angiotensin II is much more potent than angiotensin I.

3 Substance T is present in the urine. Does this *prove* that it is filterable at the glomerulus?

No. It is a possibility, but there is another; substance T may be secreted by the tubules.

4 Substance O is filtered, reabsorbed, and secreted. If you were

There are three possibilities (either alone or in combination): Increase designing a system for increasing the renal excretion of substance O when its intake is high, what could you do?

filtered substance O by increasing either GFR or plasma concentration of substance O; inhibit tubular reabsorption of substance O; enhance tubular secretion of substance O.

5 You are trying to measure the reabsorptive T_m for glucose in a patient. You plan to calculate glucose reabsorption $(C_{In} \times P_G) - (U_G \times V)$ as you raise plasma glucose stepwise by infusion. You stop the test when glucose first appears in the urine, assuming that the reabsorptive rate at this time equals the T_m. Is this correct?

No. Glucose starts to appear in the urine *before* the T_m for all nephrons has been reached. Therefore, if you had continued to raise plasma glucose, reabsorptive rate would have increased some more. You can be certain that T_m has been reached only when the reabsorptive rate remains constant despite another increment in plasma glucose.

6 A drug is given which dilates the afferent arterioles. What happens to GFR?

It increases because of an increased glomerular-capillary pressure.

7 If the concentration of protein in the glomerular filtrate was 0.005 g/100 mL and none was reabsorbed, how much protein would be excreted per day (assuming a normal GFR)?

9 g

$$\text{Excreted} = \text{filtered} - \text{reabsorbed}$$
$$= (0.05 \text{ g/L}$$
$$\times 180 \text{ L/day}) - 0$$
$$= 9 \text{ g/day}$$

8 A drug has been found to increase uric acid excretion. Give at least three ways it might act.

(1) Increase uric acid synthesis → increased plasma uric acid → increased filtration
(2) Stimulation of secretion
(3) Inhibition of reabsorption

9 If you wished to increase your patient's excretion of quinine, a weak organic base, what change in urinary pH would you try to induce?

Decreased pH. This would convert more of the quinine to its charged form and prevents its passive reabsorption.

10 The hospital lab reports that your patient's creatinine clearance is 120 g/day. This value is:
  a Normal
  b Significantly below normal
  c Nonsense

c. Clearance units are volume per time, not mass per time.

11 The following test results were obtained on specimens from a person over a 2-h period during infusion of inulin and PAH.

$$C_{In} = \frac{U_{In}V}{P_{In}}$$
$$= \frac{100 \text{ mg}/100 \text{ mL} \times 0.14 \text{ L}/2 \text{ h}}{1 \text{ mg}/100 \text{ mL}}$$
$$= 14.0 \text{ L}/2 \text{ h}; \text{ this is the GFR}$$

Total urine vol = 0.14 L
$$U_{In} = 100 \text{ mg}/100 \text{ mL}$$
$$P_{In} = 1 \text{ mg}/100 \text{ mL}$$
$$U_{urea} = 220 \text{ mmol/L}$$
$$P_{urea} = 5 \text{ mmol/L}$$
$$U_{PAH} = 700 \text{ mg/mL}$$
$$P_{PAH} = 2 \text{ mg/mL}$$
Hematocrit = 0.40

$$C_{urea} = \frac{U_{urea}V}{P_{urea}}$$
$$= \frac{220 \text{ mmol/L} \times 0.14 \text{ L}/2 \text{ h}}{5 \text{ mmol/L}}$$
$$= 6.16 \text{ L}/2 \text{ h}$$

What are the clearances of inulin, urea, and PAH? What is the effective renal plasma flow (ERPF)? What is the effective renal blood flow (ERBF)? How much urea is reabsorbed? How much PAH is secreted (assuming no PAH reabsorption and complete filterability of PAH)?

$$C_{PAH} = \frac{U_{PAH}V}{P_{PAH}}$$
$$= \frac{700 \text{ mg/mL} \times 0.14 \text{ L}/2 \text{ h}}{2 \text{ mg/mL}}$$
$$= 49.0 \text{ L}/2 \text{ h}$$

ERPF = 49.0 L/2 h
ERBF = 81.7 L/2 h

Reabsorbed
urea   = filtered urea
           − excreted urea
       = (14.0 L/2 h
           × 5 mmol/L) −
           (220 mmol/L
           × 0.14 L/2 h)
       = 39.2 mmol/2 h

PAH secreted = PAH excreted
                 − PAH filtered
           = (700 mg/mL
               × 0.14 L/2 h)
               − (2 mg/mL
               × 14.0 L/2 h)
           = 98.0 g/2 h
               − 28.0 g/2 h
           = 70.0 g/2 h

12 In the above problem, you also obtained a sample of plasma from a renal vein. Its PAH concentration was 0.2 mg/mL. What is the true renal plasma flow?

$$TRPF = \frac{U_{PAH}V}{P_{PAH} - \text{renal venous}_{PAH}} =$$
$$\frac{700 \text{ mg/mL} \times 0.14 \text{ L}/2 \text{ h}}{2 \text{ mg/mL} - 0.2 \text{ mg/mL}}$$
$$= 54.4 \text{ L}/2 \text{ h}$$

13 Now that you know that the renal venous plasma contained PAH, was the value you calculated for secreted PAH the secretory T_m for PAH?

No. There is always PAH in the renal venous plasma, mainly because some of the renal blood flow does not pass near proximal tubules. The way to do a PAH secretory T_m is to keep raising the systemic plasma PAH by infusion and when the mass of PAH secreted (calculated just as you did in the problem) stops increasing with further increments in systemic plasma PAH, that mass is the T_m.

14 An increase in the plasma concentration of inulin causes which of the following in the renal clearance of inulin:
  a   Increase
  b   Decrease
  c   No change

c. $C_{In} = U_{In}V/P_{In}$. When P_{In} increases, there is no change in C_{In} because U_{In} rises an identical amount. In other words, the mass of inulin filtered and excreted increases but the volume of plasma supplying this inulin, i.e., completely cleared of inulin, is unaltered.

15 The clearance of substance A is less than that simultaneously determined for inulin. Give three possible explanations.

(1) Substance A is, itself, a large molecule poorly filtered at the glomerulus.
(2) Substance A is bound, at least in part, to plasma protein.
(3) Substance A is reabsorbed.

16 List in order of decreasing renal clearance the following substances:
  Glucose
  Urea
  Sodium
  Inulin
  Creatinine
  PAH

PAH
Creatinine
Inulin
Urea
Sodium
Glucose

17 If 50 percent of the nephrons were destroyed, which of the following compounds would be likely to show an increased blood concentration?
  a   Urea

a, b, c. These waste products are all normally excreted in large amounts; a decreased GFR would cause their plasma concentrations to increase until filtered load was increased enough to reestablish

b   Creatinine
c   Uric acid
d   Most amino acids
e   Glucose
f   Purines

normal excretion. In contrast, the reabsorption T_m's for glucose, amino acids, purines, and many other organic compounds which are not waste products are usually so high as to prevent significant excretion. Accordingly, their plasma concentrations are virtually independent of renal function; i.e., the kidneys do not participate in the setting of their plasma concentrations.

18 A month after 80 percent of the nephrons are destroyed, what will the blood-urea concentration be, assuming it was 5 mmol/L before the disease occurred.
a   25 mmol/L
b   5 mmol/L
c   6 mmol/L
d   Continuously rising
e   Not calculable unless it is assumed that the patient's protein intake did not change as a result of the disease

e. If one assumes a constant protein intake, then 25 mmol/L would have been the correct answer, since total filtered urea could be restored to normal at this point [25(0.2 × 180) = 5 × 180]. However, had protein intake been reduced by 50 percent, then plasma urea would stabilize at 12.5 mmol/L, since only 50 percent as much urea would be produced.

19 During a dog experiment, a clamp around the renal artery is partially tightened so as to reduce renal arterial pressure from a mean of 120 mmHg to 80 mmHg. How much do you predict RBF will change?
a   33 percent decrease
b   Zero
c   5 to 10 percent decrease
d   33 percent increase

c. Autoregulation prevents the RBF from decreasing in direct proportion to mean arterial pressure, but autoregulation is not 100 percent.

20 A patient suffers a hemorrhage which drops the mean arterial pressure by 25 percent. What do you predict happens to the GFR and RBF?
a   Almost no change

b. If you answered "a," you probably assumed that autoregulation would prevent any significant change. This is wrong because the drop in pressure reflexly stimulates increased sympathetic tone to the

b A fairly large decrease, RBF > GFR

kidney. (See text for the reason the GFR change is less than the RBF change.)

21 In the steady state, what is the amount of sodium chloride excreted daily in the urine by a normal person ingesting 12 g of sodium chloride per day?
  a 12 g/day
  b Less than 12 g/day

b. Urinary excretion in the steady state must be less than ingested sodium chloride by an amount equal to that lost in the sweat and feces. This is normally quite small, less than 1 g/day, so that urine excretion in this case equals approximately 11 g/day.

22 A person's plasma sodium concentration is 144 mmol/L, inulin clearance, 120 mL/min; urine volume, 36 mL in 30 min; and the urine sodium concentration, 200 mmol/L. What percent of filtered sodium is excreted?

1.4%
$$\text{Filtered Na}^+ = 144 \text{ mmol/L}$$
$$\times\ 0.12 \text{ L/min}$$
$$= 17.28 \text{ mmol/min}$$
$$\text{Excreted Na}^+ = 0.036 \text{ L/}$$
$$30 \text{ min} \times$$
$$200 \text{ mmol/L}$$
$$= 0.24 \text{ mmol/min}$$
$$\%\ \frac{\text{Excreted}}{\text{Filtered}} = \frac{0.24}{17.28}$$
$$\times\ 100 = 1.4\%$$

23 In chronic renal disease plasma urea may become markedly elevated. Under such circumstances urea will act as an osmotic diuretic. What does this do to sodium, chloride, and water excretion?

Sodium, chloride, and water excretion will all increase.

24 Normally there are no *passive* fluxes of sodium into or out of the proximal tubule. True or false?

False. There are very large passive fluxes in both directions. However, there is little *net* flux because of the absence of a significant electrochemical gradient for sodium.

25a Complete inhibition of active chloride transport by the ascending loop of Henle would virtually eliminate the ability to excrete a concentrated urine. True or false?
  b Increasing the passive permeability of the ascending loop to

(*a*) True.
(*b*) True. The gradient between ascending loop and interstitium at any *horizontal* level would be decreased; therefore the gradient from top to bottom would be decreased.

chloride would reduce the maximal concentrating ability of the kidney. True or false?

c Active reabsorption of sodium by the descending loop is a component of the countercurrent multiplier system. True or false?

(c) False. There is no reabsorption of sodium (or chloride) by the descending loop.

26 A normal experimental animal is given a drug, and a sample of tubular fluid (TF) is later collected by micropuncture from the end of the proximal convoluted tubule along with a plasma (P) sample. The TF/P ratio for inulin is 1.5 and for sodium is 0.99. Has the drug inhibited, stimulated, or done nothing to proximal sodium reabsorption?

Inhibited it. The inulin data reveal that only 30 percent of filtered water has been reabsorbed. Since TF/P for sodium is essentially unity (the normal value for proximal fluid), this means that only 30 percent of the filtered sodium was reabsorbed, a value far below normal.

27 True or false questions.

a Net reabosrption of sodium occurs in the ascending loop of Henle.

b Net reabsorption of water occurs in the descending loop.

c Net reabsorption of water occurs in the collecting ducts.

d Net bulk flow of interstitial fluid into the vasa recta occurs.

All are true. The last may have given you trouble. The fact is that the vasa recta act as countercurrent exchangers to eliminate net overall *diffusion* of sodium and water into or out of the vasa recta by balancing any net movements in the descending vessels with opposite ones in the ascending. Thus, net diffusional movements are minimal, but normal capillary *bulk flow* must still be occurring, or otherwise the sodium and water reabsorbed from the loops of Henle and collecting duct would not be carried away.

28 In an experiment a dog's rate of glomerular filtration of sodium is found to be 15 mmol/min.

a How much sodium do you predict remains in the tubule at the end of the proximal tubule?

b Its GFR is suddenly in-

(a) 5 mmol/min. Approximately two-thirds of filtered sodium is reabsorbed by the proximal tubule.

(b) 6.6 mmol/min. Filtered sodium rises from 15 to 20 mmol/min. Glomerulotubular balance maintains fractional sodium reabsorp-

creased by 33 percent. How much sodium now is left at the end of the proximal tubule?

tion at approximately two-thirds of the filtered load.

29 Normally aldosterone controls the reabsorption of approximately 33 g of sodium chloride per day. If a patient loses 100 percent of adrenal function, will 33 g of sodium chloride be excreted per day indefinitely?

No. As soon as the patient starts to become sodium-deficient as a result of the increased sodium excretion, the usual sodium-retaining reflexes will be set into motion. They will, of course, be unable to raise aldosterone secretion, but they will lower GFR and alter the other factors which influence tubular sodium reabsorption so as to at least partially compensate for the decreased aldosterone-dependent sodium reabsorption.

30 What happens to sodium excretion during quiet standing?

It decreases. Because of venous pooling of blood and increased filtration of fluid across the leg capillaries, quiet standing causes an effective decrease in plasma volume, which triggers all the described inputs leading to decreased sodium excretion (decreased GFR and increased tubular reabsorption).

31 A patient has just suffered a severe hemorrhage and the plasma protein concentration is normal. (Not enough time has elapsed for interstitial fluid to move into the plasma.) Does this mean that the peritubular-capillary oncotic pressure is also normal?

No. It will probably be above normal because of an increased filtration fraction secondary to sympathetically mediated renal arteriolar constriction.

32 If the right renal artery becomes abnormally constricted, what will happen to renin secretion by it and by the left kidney?

The right kidney has an increased secretion because of the decreased renal perfusion acting via the intra-renal baroreceptor and macula densa. This increased secretion will result in elevated systemic angiotensin and arterial blood pressure, both of which will inhibit renin secretion from the left kidney.

33 A patient with leaky glomeruli but normal tubules loses protein in the urine and, therefore, has a plasma albumin of 2.5 g/100 mL. Virtually all sodium ingested is retained (i.e., urinary excretion of sodium is close to zero) and the patient is becoming edematous. What is the stimulus for renal sodium retention in this case, since total extracellular volume is clearly greater than normal?

Because of the low plasma albumin, *plasma volume is decreased* as a result of the abnormal balance of forces across capillaries. This decreased plasma volume initiated sodium-retaining reflexes just as if the plasma volume had been decreased by diarrhea, a burn, etc. The retained fluid does not restore the plasma volume to normal, however, but merely filters into the interstitium, where it increases the edema. Interestingly, tubular sodium reabsorption is increased in this state despite the fact that peritubular-capillary protein concentration is almost certainly lower than normal, which should reduce tubular sodium reabsorption. A reflexly increased aldosterone level is certainly important in stimulating sodium reabsorption and overriding this effect of the low protein. Changes in renal hemodynamics and in the postulated natriuretic hormone may also be important.

34 A patient is suffering from primary hyperaldosteronism, i.e., increased secretion of aldosterone, usually caused by an aldosterone-producing adrenal tumor. Is plasma renin concentration higher or lower than normal?

Lower. The increased aldosterone causes positive sodium balance, which reflexly inhibits renin secretion. Thus, one observes a high plasma aldosterone and a low plasma renin—a strong tip-off as to the presence of the disease, since in almost all other situations renin and aldosterone change in the same direction (because renin-angiotensin is the major control of aldosterone secretion).

35 Any agent which increases sodium and water excretion is called a diuretic (even though natriuretic is probably a better term). List pos-

(1) Increase GFR either by raising blood pressure or by dilating renal afferent arterioles.
(2)   The   above   hemodynamic

sible mechanisms of actions of these drugs.

changes would also inhibit sodium reabsorption by increasing peritubular-capillary hydraulic pressure and/or reducing peritubular-capillary oncotic pressure (because of decreased filtration fraction).
(3) Directly inhibit the active-transport system for sodium, e.g., by blocking its energy supply, or for chloride (in the loop).
(4) Inhibit secretion of renin or aldosterone.
(5) Block action of aldosterone.
(6) Act as an osmotic diuretic by its osmotic contribution (mannitol, for example).
(7) Inhibit active secretory system for hydrogen (e.g., by blocking carbonic anhydrase). (You will not know this now, but will by the end of the book.)

This list is by no means exhaustive but does include the major clinically useful types of diuretics.

36 A normal subject loses 2 L of isotonic salt solution because of diarrhea. He or she simultaneously drinks 2 L of pure water. What happens to:
   a Extracellular-fluid volume
   b Body-fluid osmolarity
   c Renin and aldosterone secretion
   d ADH secretion

(*a*) and (*b*) Extracellular volume and osmolarity both decrease. The entire 2 L of solution was lost from the extracellular compartment, since it was isotonic. (Therefore, osmolarity did not change, and no water moved into or out of cells.) The 2 L of ingested pure water is distributed throughout the body water, only about one-third remaining in the extracellular fluid. Moreover, the addition of pure water lowers the osmolarity.
(*c*) Increases, because of reflexes induced by the decreased extracellular volume.
(*d*) Cannot predict for certain but probably decreases. The decreased extracellular volume reflexly stimu-

lates ADH secretion, but the reduced osmolarity should inhibit it via the hypothalamic osmoreceptors. The osmoreceptor input usually predominates during such "conflicts" unless the extracellular-volume depletion is very large.

37 A person excretes 2 L of urine having an osmolarity of 600 mosmol/L. As a result, does body-fluid osmolarity *increase* or *decrease?* The change would be identical to that produced by *adding or subtracting how many* liters of pure water?

Decrease; adding 2 L. He or she has excreted 2 L × 600 mosmol/L = 1200 mosmol total solute and 2 L water. Two liters of normal body fluids contain 2 L × 300 mosmol/L = 600 mosmol solutes. Accordingly, he or she has excreted 1200 − 600 = 600 mosmol pure solute beyond that needed for isotonicity. This will reduce the body-fluid osmolarity by an amount equivalent to that produced by adding 2 L pure water; i.e., 2 L of "free water" are retained.

38 A person excreted 3 L of urine having an osmolarity of 150 mosmol/L. As a result, does body-fluid osmolarity *increase* or *decrease?* The change is identical to that produced by *adding or subtracting how many* liters pure water to/or from the body?

Increase; subtracting 1.5 L. He or she has excreted 3 L × 150 mosmol/L = 450 mosmol total solute, and 3 L water have been excreted. This amount of solute is contained in 450 mosmol ÷ 300 mosmol/L = 1.5 L normal body fluid. Therefore he or she has excreted 3 L − 1.5 L = 1.5 L "free water" from the body, thereby raising its osmolarity.

39 What are the major renal sites of action of the following hormones?
Aldosterone
ADH
Renin
Epinephrine

Aldosterone: Distal tubule and collecting duct
ADH: Distal tubule and collecting duct
Renin: No renal site of action
Epinephrine: Renal arterioles, JG apparatus, and renal tubules

40 What are the major controls of aldosterone secretion rate?

(1) Angiotensin
(2) ACTH
(3) Plasma sodium concentration
(4) Plasma potassium concentration

41 What are the major controls of renin secretion?

(1) Afferent-arteriolar pressure (intrarenal-baroreceptor)
(2) Sodium chloride load to the macula densa
(3) Activity of renal sympathetic nerves
(4) Angiotensin

42 What are the major controls of ADH secretion?

(1) Body-fluid osmolarity via hypothalamic osmoreceptors (or Na receptors)
(2) Plasma volume (specifically left atrial pressure via baroreceptors)

43 Control of potassium excretion is achieved mainly by regulating the rate of:
  a Potassium filtration
  b Potassium reabsorption
  c Potassium secretion

c

44 A person in previously normal potassium balance maintains neurotic hyperventilation for several days. During this period what happens to potassium balance?

It becomes negative. The hyperventilation causes alkalosis, which in turn induces increased secretion of potassium (probably due to an alkalosis-induced elevation of renal-tubular-cell potassium concentration).

45 A patient has a tumor in the adrenal which continuously secretes large quantities of aldosterone (primary hyperaldosteronism). Is the rate of potassium excretion normal, high, or low?

High. The increased aldosterone stimulates potassium secretion and, thereby, excretion. Moreover, once enough sodium has been retained to cause partial inhibition of proximal and loop sodium reabsorption, the increased delivery of fluid to the distal nephron further enhances potassium secretion. There is no potassium escape similar to the sodium escape from aldosterone.

46 A patient with severe congestive heart failure is secreting large quantities of aldosterone. Is the rate of potassium excretion normal, high, or low?

Relatively normal. You may well have answered "high" assuming that the increased aldosterone would stimulate potassium secretion, as in the previous question.

However, this effect is more than balanced by the fact that the patient has a diminished flow of fluid into the distal tubule (because of increased proximal and loop reabsorption); recall that potassium secretion is greatly impaired when the amount of fluid flowing through the distal tubule is reduced. This explains why patients with the diseases of secondary hyperaldosteronism with edema do not lose large quantities of potassium, whereas patients with primary hyperaldosteronism do.

47 Give three reasons why osmotic diuresis (as, for example, in uncontrolled diabetic ketoacidosis) enhances potassium excretion.

(1) It inhibits potassium reabsorption.
(2) It increases fluid delivery to the distal tubule, resulting in increased potassium secretion.
(3) It causes sodium depletion, which increases aldosterone secretion (via the renin-angiotensin system), and this hormone stimulates potassium secretion.

48 A patient is observed to excrete 2 L of alkaline (pH = 7.6) urine having a bicarbonate concentration of 28 mmol/L. The rate of titratable-acid excretion is:
   a   56 mmol
   b   Negative
   c   Cannot tell without data for ammonium

b. If the urine has a pH greater than 7.4, then clearly there is no titratable acid (t.a.) excreted; indeed, there is negative t.a. excretion. Ammonium does not contribute to t.a. and may be ignored in the calculation of t.a.

49 The following data are obtained for a subject:
$$C_{In} = 170 \text{ L/day}$$
$$P_{HCO_3^-} = 25 \text{ mmol/L}$$
$$U_{HCO_3^-} = 0$$
Urine pH = 5.8
Titratable acid = 26 mmol/day
Urine NH_4^+ = 48 mmol/day

(a) 4324 mmol/day. (Sum of HCO_3^- reabsorbed, t.a. excreted, and NH_4^+ excreted.)
(b) 74 mmol/day. (Sum of t.a. and NH_4^+.)

Calculate:

  a Total hydrogen ion secreted

  b New bicarbonate added to the blood, i.e., acid excreted

50 Which values could you predict are those for a patient with primary hyperaldosteronism?

	Urine pH	Plasma pH
a	6.9	7.55
b	8.2	7.55
c	4.8	7.30

a. This patient secretes excessive amounts of aldosterone, which induces potassium deficiency (because of increased renal potassium secretion). The potassium deficiency and aldosterone together then induce inappropriately large renal hydrogen-ion secretion, thereby producing a metabolic alkalosis. Note that the urine is still acid; i.e., the kidneys are not compensating.

51 A patient has been losing large amounts of HCl because of persistent vomiting for 3 days and, therefore, has a plasma pH of 7.50. The urine pH was 8.0 at the end of day one and 6.9 at the end of day three. Explain.

The alkaline urine on day one is the appropriate renal compensation for vomiting-induced alkalosis. The slightly acid urine on day three signifies that the kidneys are no longer compensating for alkalosis. This happens mainly because the progressive development of severe salt depletion stimulates proximal hydrogen-ion secretion, preventing loss of bicarbonate in the urine. (Potassium depletion and increased aldosterone may also contribute.)

52 If renal tubular carbonic anhydrase were completely inhibited, you would expect increased excretion of which of the following?

  a Sodium
  b Water
  c Chloride
  d Bicarbonate
  e Ammonium
  f Potassium

a, b, d, and f. See text for explanation of these increases. If anything, chloride excretion will decrease because of the reciprocal relationship between bicarbonate and reabsorption. Ammonium excretion will be close to nil because the alkalinity of the tubular fluid minimizes diffusion trapping of ammonia.

53 Match the top column with
the bottom column. ("Increased"
or "decreased" is with reference
to normal.)

(a) 2
(b) 3
(c) 1

   a Diabetic ketoacidosis
   b Hypoventilation
   c Excessive ingestion of sodium bicarbonate
   1. Increased plasma pH, increased plasma bicarbonate, alkaline urine
   2. Decreased plasma pH, decreased plasma bicarbonate, acidic
urine
   3. Decreased plasma pH, increased plasma bicarbonate, acidic
urine

54 Which of the following would
you expect to find in a patient suffering from primary hypersecretion of parathyroid hormone?
   a Increased plasma calcium
   b Decreased plasma phosphate
   c Increased urine calcium
   d Increased tubular reabsorption of calcium
   e Increased urine phosphate
   f Increased plasma calcitonin
   g Increased plasma
$1,25\text{-}(OH)_2D_3$

All are correct. c and d are not
mutually exclusive because of the
marked increase in filtered calcium. Calcitonin is reflexly increased
by the increased plasma calcium.
Formation of $1,25\text{-}(OH)_2D_3$ is enhanced by parathyroid hormone
and by the decreased plasma
phosphate as well.

55 Complete inhibition of active
sodium reabsorption would cause
an increase in the excretion of
which of the following substances?
   a Water
   b Urea
   c Chloride
   d Glucose
   e Amino acids
   f Potassium
   g Bicarbonate
   h Calcium

All. The reasons are all given in
relevant sections of the text.

Suggested Readings

RESEARCH TECHNIQUES

Burg, M., and J. Orloff: Perfusion of Isolated Renal Tubules, in R. W. Berliner and J. Orloff (eds.), "Handbook of Renal Physiology," sec. 8, American Physiological Society, Wash., D.C., 1973.

Gottschalk, C. W., and W. E. Lassiter: Micropuncture Methodology, in R. W. Berliner and J. Orloff (eds.), "Handbook of Renal Physiology," sec. 8, American Physiological Society, Wash., D.C., 1973.

Levinsky, N. G., and M. Levy: Clearance Techniques, in R. W. Berliner and J. Orloff (eds.), "Handbook of Renal Physiology," sec. 8, American Physiological Society, Wash., D.C., 1973.

Malvin, R. L., and W. S. Wilde: Stop-flow Technique, in R. W. Berliner, and J. Orloff (eds.), "Handbook of Renal Physiology," sec. 8, American Physiological Society, Wash., D.C., 1973.

CHAP. 1

Anderson, R. J. et al.: Prostaglandins, *Kidney Int.,* **10:**205 (1976).

Barger, A. C., and J. A. Herd: Renal Vascular Anatomy and Distribution of Blood Flow, in R. W. Berliner and J. Orloff (eds.), "Handbook of Renal Physiology," sec. 8, American Physiological Society, Wash., D.C., 1973.

Beeuwkes, R., and J. V. Boventre: Tubular Organization and Vascular-tubular Relations in the Dog Kidney, *Am. J. Physiol.*, **229:**695 (1975). Read this to see how complex the anatomy really is.

Dalton, A. J., and F. Hagenau (eds.): "Ultrastructure of the Kidney," Academic, New York, 1967.

Oliver, J.: "Nephrons and Kidneys: A Quantitative Study of Developmental and Evolutionary Mammalian Architectonics," Harper & Row, New York, 1968.

Peach, M. J.: Renin-Angiotensin System: Biochemistry and Mechanisms of Action, *Physiol. Res.*, **57:**313 (1977).

Rouiller, C., and A. F. Muller (eds.): "The Kidney," vol. 1, Academic, New York, 1969.

Tisher, C. C.: Functional Anatomy of the Kidney, *Hosp. Pract.*, May (1978).

Wright, F. S.: Sites and Mechanisms of Potassium Transport along the Renal Tubule, *Kidney Int.*, **11:**415 (1977).

CHAP. 2

Brenner, B. M., and T. H. Hostetter.: Molecular Basis of Proteinuria of Glomerular Origin, *N. Engl. J. Med.*, **298:**826 (1978).

Brenner, B. M., and H. D. Humes.: Mechanics of Glomerular Ultrafiltration, *N. Engl. J. Med.*, **297:**148 (1977).

Deen, W. M., C. R. Robertson, and B. M. Brenner: Glomerular Ultrafiltration, *Fed. Proc.*, **33:**14 (1974). The most concise review of glomerular pressures and the dependence of GFR on RBF.

Hayes, R. M.: Principles of Ion and Water Transport in the Kidney, *Hosp. Pract.*, Sept. (1978).

Hopfer, U.: Transport in Isolated Plasma Membranes, *Am. J. Physiol.*, **234:**F89 (1978).

Kassirer, J. P.: Clinical Evaluation of Kidney Function–Tubular Function, *N. Engl. J. Med.*, **285:**499 (1971).

Pappenheimer, J. R.: Passage of Molecules through Capillary Walls, *Physiol. Rev.*, **33:**387 (1953). A discussion of the basic concepts and principles of ultrafiltration.

Pitts, R. F.: "Physiology of the Kidney and Body Fluids," 3d ed., chaps. 6 and 8, Year Book, Chicago, 1974. General descriptions of tubular reabsorption and secretion. This is also a good source of information on the transport systems for specific substances (glucose, phosphate, etc.).

Renkin, E. M., and J. Gilmore: Glomerular Filtration, in R. W. Berliner and J. Orloff (eds.), "Handbook of Renal Physiology," sec. 8, American Physiological Society, Wash., D.C., 1973.

Renkin, E. M., and R. R. Robinson: Glomerular Filtration, *N. Engl. J. Med.*, **290:**785 (1974).

CHAP. 3

Burg, M. B.: The Nephron in Transport of Sodium, Amino Acids, and Glucose, *Hosp. Pract.*, Oct. (1978).

Lassiter, W. E.: Uric Acid Excretion, *Annu. Rev. Physiol.*, **37:**385 (1975).

Maunsbach, A. B.: Cellular Mechanisms of Tubular Protein Transport, in "Kidney and Urinary Tract Physiology II," International Review of Physiology, vol. 11, University Park Press, Baltimore, 1976.

Ullrich, K. J.: Renal Tubular Mechanisms of Organic Solute Transport, *Kidney Int.*, **9:**134 (1976).

CHAP. 4

Kassirer, J. P.: Clinical Evaluation of Kidney Function–Glomerular Function, *N. Engl. J. Med.*, **285:**385 (1971).

Levinsky, N. G., and M. Levy: Clearance Techniques, in R. W. Berliner and J. Orloff (eds.), "Handbook of Renal Physiology," sec. 8, American Physiological Society, Wash., D.C., 1973.

Smith, H. W.: "Principles of Renal Physiology," chaps. 3–6, Oxford, New York, 1956.

CHAP. 5

Barger, A. C., and J. A. Herd: Renal Vascular Anatomy and Distribution of Blood Flow, in R. W. Berliner and J. Orloff (eds.), "Handbook of Renal Physiology," sec. 8, American Physiological Society, Wash., D.C., 1973.

Brenner, B. M., and R. Beeuwkes III: The Renal Circulations, *Hosp. Pract.*, July (1978).

Deen, W. M., C. R. Robertson, and B. M. Brenner: Glomerular Ultrafiltration, *Fed. Proc.*, **33:**14 (1974).

Dunn, M. J., and V. L. Hood: Prostaglandins and the Kidney, *Am. J. Physiol.*, **232:**F169 (1967).

Johnson, P. C. (ed.): Autoregulation of Blood Flow, *Circ. Res.*, vol. 15, supplement I, 1964, pp. 103–200.

Navar, G. L.: Renal Autoregulation: Perspectives from Whole Kidney and Single Nephron Studies, *Am. J. Physiol.*, **234:**F357 (1978).

Needleman, P., et al.: Determinants and Modification of Adrenergic and Vascular Resistance in the Kidney, *Am. J. Physiol.*, **227:**665 (1974).

Selkurt, E. E.: The Renal Circulation, in W. I. Hamilton and P. Dow, "Handbook of Physiology," sec. 2, vol. II, American Physiological Society, Wash., D.C., 1963.

Tucker, B. J., and R. C. Blantz: An Analysis of the Determinants of Nephron Filtration Rate, *Am. J. Physiol.*, **232:**F477 (1977).

Wright, Fred S.: Intrarenal Regulation of Glomerular Filtration Rate, *N. Engl. J. Med.*, **291:**135 1(974).

CHAP. 6

Andreolli, T. E., R. W. Berliner, J. P. Kokko, and D. J. Marsh: Questions and Replies: Renal Mechanisms for Urinary Concentrating and Diluting Processes, *Am. J. Physiol.*, **235:**F1 (1978).

Andreolli, T. E., and J. A. Schafer: Effective Luminal Hypotonicity: The Driving Force for Isotonic Proximal Tubular Fluid Absorption, *Am. J. Physiol.,* **236:**F89 (1979).

Boulpaep, E. L.: Recent Advances in Electrophysiology of the Nephron, *Annu. Rev. Physiol.,* **38:**20 (1976).

Burg, M. B.: The Nephron in Transport of Sodium, Amino Acids, and Glucose, *Hosp. Pract.,* Oct. (1978).

Burg, M. B., and J. Orloff: Perfusion of Isolated Renal Tubules, in R. W. Berliner and J. Orloff (eds.), "Handbook of Renal Physiology," sec. 8, American Physiological Society, Wash., D.C., 1973.

Dousa, T. P., and H. Valtin: Cellular Actions of Vasopressin in the Mammalian Kidney, *Kidney Int.,* **10:**46 (1976).

Giebisch, G., and E. Windhager: Electrolyte Transport Across Renal Tubular Membranes, in R. W. Berliner and J. Orloff (eds.), "Handbook of Renal Physiology," sec. 8, American Physiological Society, Wash., D.C., 1973.

Grantham, J. J., J. M. Irish III, and D. A. Hall: Studies of Isolated Renal Tubules in Vitro, *Am. Rev. Physiol.,* **40:**249 (1978).

Kokko, J. P.: Membrane Characteristics Governing Salt and Water Transport in the Loop of Henle, *Fed. Proc.,* **33:**25 (1974).

Kokko, J. P.: Renal Concentrating and Diluting Mechanisms, *Hosp. Pract.,* Feb. (1979).

Sachs, G.: Ion Pumps in the Renal Tubule, *Am. J. Physiol.,* **235:**F359 (1977).

Stoff, J. S., et al.: Recent Advances in Renal Tubular Biochemistry, *Annu. Rev. Physiol.,* **38:**46 (1976).

CHAP. 7

Andersson, B.: Regulation of Body Fluids, *Annu. Rev. Physiol.,* **39:**185 (1977).

Andersson, B.: Regulation of Water Intake, *Physiol. Rev.,* **58:**582 (1978).

Brenner, B. M., and J. L. Troy: Postglomerular Vascular Protein Concentration: Evidence for a Causal Role in Governing Fluid Reabsorption and Glomerulotubular Balance by the Renal Proximal Tubule, *J. Clin. Invest.,* **50:**336 (1971).

Cannon, P. J.: The Kidney in Heart Failure, *N. Engl. J. Med.,* **296:**26 (1977).

Davis, J. O.: The Control of Renin Release, *Am. J. Med.,* **55:**333 (1973).

Denton, D. A.: Salt Appetite, in C. F. Code and W. Heidel (eds.), "Handbook of Physiology," sec. 6, vol. I, American Physiological Society, 1967.

De Wardener, H. E.: The Control of Sodium Excretion, *Am. J. Physiol.,* **235:**F163 (1978).

DiBona, G. F.: Neural Control of Renal Tubular Sodium Reabsorption in the Dog, *Fed. Proc.,* **37:**1214 (1978).

Dunn, M. J., and V. L. Hood: Prostaglandins and the Kidney, *Am. J. Physiol.,* **233:**F169 (1977).

Earley, L. E., and R. W. Schrier: Intrarenal Control of Sodium Excretion by Hemodynamic and Physical Factors, in R. W. Berliner and J. Orloff (eds.), "Handbook of Renal Physiology," sec. 8, American Physiological Society, Wash., D.C., 1973.

Gauer, D. H., and J. P. Henry: Circulatory Basis of Fluid Volume Control, *Physiol. Rev.,* **43:**423 (1963).

Jacobson, H. R., and D. W. Seldin: Proximal Tubular Reabsorption and Its Regulation, *Annu. Rev. Pharm. Toxicol.,* **17:**623 (1977).

Laragh, J. H., and J. E. Sealey: The Renin-Angiotensin-Aldosterone Hormonal System and Regulation of Sodium, Potassium, and Blood Pressure Homeostasis, in R. W. Berliner and J. Orloff (eds.), "Handbook of Renal Physiology," sec. 8, American Physiological Society, Wash., D.C., 1973.

Lemeire, N. H., M. D. Lifschitz, and J. H. Stein: Heterogenicity of Nephron Function, *Annu. Rev. Physiol.,* **39:**159 (1977).

Oparil, S., and E. Haber: The Renin-Angiotensin System, *N. Engl. J. Med.,* **291:**389 (1974).

Reid, I. A., B. J. Morris, and W. F. Ganong: The Renin-Angiotensin System, *Annu. Rev. Physiol.,* **40:**377 (1978).

Robertson, G. L., R. L. Shelton, and S. Atkar: The Osmoregulation of Vasopressin, *Kidney Int.,* **10:**25 (1976).

Schrier, R. W., and T. Berl: Nonosmolar Factors Affecting Renal Water Excretion, *N. Engl. J. Med.,* **292:**81 (1975).

Smith, H. W.: Salt and Water Volume Receptors, *Am. J. Med.,* **23:**623 (1957).

Stein, J. H., and H. J. Reineck: The Role of the Collecting Duct in the Regulation of Excretion of Sodium and Other Electrolytes, *Kidney Int.,* **6:**1 (1974).

Windhager, E. E.: Some Aspects of Proximal Tubular Salt Reabsorption, *Fed. Proc.,* **33:**21 (1974). A concise review of the role of peritubular pressures in sodium reabsorption.

CHAP. 8

Gennari, F. J., and J. J. Cohen: Role of the Kidney in Potassium Homeostasis: Lessons from Acid-Base Disturbances, *Kidney Int.,* **8:**1 (1975). Attempts to explain the mechanisms by which potassium excretion is influenced by acid-base disturbances.

Knochel, J. P.: Role of Glucoregulatory Hormones in Potassium Homeostasis, *Kidney Int.,* **11:**443 (1977).

Macknight, A. D. C.: Epithelial Transport of Potassium, *Kidney Int.,* **11:**391 (1977). Describes problems in the classic model for transepithelial transport.

Silva, P., R. S. Brown, and F. H. Epstein: Adaptation to Potassium, *Kidney Int.,* **11:**466 (1977).

Stein, J. H., and H. J. Reineck: The Role of the Collecting Duct in the Regulation and Excretion of Sodium and Other Electrolytes, *Kidney Int.,* **6:**1 (1974).

Wright, F. S.: Sites and Mechanisms of Potassium Transport along the Renal Tubule, *Kidney Int.,* **11:**415 (1977).

Wright, F. S., and G. Giebisch: Renal Potassium Transport: Contributions of Different Nephron Segments and Populations, *Am. J. Physiol.,* **235:**F515 (1978).

CHAP. 9

Arruda, J. A. L., and N. A. Kurtzman: Relationship of Renal Sodium and Water Transport to Hydrogen Ion Secretion, *Annu. Rev. Physiol.,* **40:**43 (1978).

Giebisch, G., and G. Malnic: Studies on the Mechanism of Tubular Acidification, *The Physiologist,* **19:**511 (1976).

Malnic, G., and P. R. Steinmetz: Transport Processes in Urinary Acidification, *Kidney Int.,* **9:**172 (1976).

Maren, T. B.: Chemistry of the Renal Reabsorption of Bicarbonate, *Can. J. Biochem. Physiol.,* **52:**1041 (1974).

Pitts, R. F.: Production and Excretion of Ammonia in Relation to Acid-Base Regulation, in R. W. Berliner and J. Orloff (eds.), "Handbook of Renal Physiology," sec. 8, American Physiological Society, Wash., D.C., 1973.

Rector, F. C., Jr.: Acidification of the Urine, in R. W. Berliner and J. Orloff (eds.), "Handbook of Renal Physiology," sec. 8, American Physiological Society, Wash., D.C., 1973.

Schwartz, W. B., C. Van Ypersele de Strihou, and J. P. Kassirer: Role of Anions in Metabolic Alkalosis and Potassium Deficiency, *N. Engl. J. Med.,* **279:**630 (1968).

Seldin, D. W., and F. C. Rector, Jr.: The Generation and Maintenance of Metabolic Alkalosis, *Kidney Int.,* **1:**306 (1972).

Steinmetz, P. R.: Cellular Mechanisms of Urinary Acidification, *Physiol. Rev.,* **54:**890 (1974).

Tannen, R. L.: Ammonia Metabolism, *Am. J. Physiol.,* **235:**F265 (1978).

CHAP. 10

Aurbach, G. D., and D. A. Heath: Parathyroid Hormone and Calcitonin Regulation of Renal Function, *Kidney Int.,* **6:**331 (1974).

DeLucca, H. F.: The Kidney as an Endocrine Organ for the Production of 1,25-dihydroxyvitamin D_3, a Calcium-mobilizing Hormone, *N. Engl. J. Med.,* **289:**359 (1973).

Goldberg, M., Z. S. Agus, and S. Goldfarb: Renal Handling of Calcium and Phosphate, in "Kidney and Urinary Tract Physiology II," *Int. Rev. Physiol.,* vol. 11, University Park Press, Baltimore, 1976.

Haussler, M. R., and T. A. McCain: Basic and Clinical Concepts Related to Vitamin D Metabolism and Action, *N. Engl. J. Med.* **297:**974 and 1041 (1977).

Massry, S. G., and J. W. Coburn: The Hormonal and Non-hormonal Control of Renal Excretion of Calcium and Magnesium, *Nephron,* **10:**66 (1973).

Walser, M.: Divalent Cations: Physicochemical State in Glomerular Filtrate and Urine and Renal Excretion, in R. W. Berliner and J. Orloff (eds.), "Handbook of Renal Physiology," sec. 8, American Physiological Society, Wash., D.C., 1973.

STAYING UP-TO-DATE

The most painless way to follow important developments in renal physiology is to read the excellent reviews which appear frequently in the *New England Journal of Medicine* and *Hospital Practice.* They are usually succinct and emphasize the clinical implications of new research findings. More detailed reviews are to be found in the Annual Review of Physiology and in the specialty journals for renal physiology, notably the *American Journal of Physiology* (Renal and Electrolyte Section) and *Kidney International.*

Index